Clinical Trials in Oncology
Third Edition

CHAPMAN & HALL/CRC
Interdisciplinary Statistics Series

Series editors: N. Keiding, B.J.T. Morgan, C.K. Wikle, P. van der Heijden

Published titles

Published titles

Chapman & Hall/CRC
Interdisciplinary Statistics Series

Clinical Trials in Oncology

Third Edition

Stephanie Green   Angela Smith
Jacqueline Benedetti   John Crowley

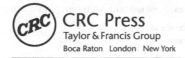

CRC Press
Taylor & Francis Group
Boca Raton   London   New York

CRC Press is an imprint of the
Taylor & Francis Group, an **informa** business

A CHAPMAN & HALL BOOK

CRC Press
Taylor & Francis Group
6000 Broken Sound Parkway NW, Suite 300
Boca Raton, FL 33487-2742

First issued in paperback 2016

© 2012 by Taylor & Francis Group, LLC
CRC Press is an imprint of Taylor & Francis Group, an Informa business

No claim to original U.S. Government works

ISBN 13: 978-1-138-19911-8 (pbk)
ISBN 13: 978-1-4398-1448-2 (hbk)

**Visit the Taylor & Francis Web site at
http://www.taylorandfrancis.com**

**and the CRC Press Web site at
http://www.crcpress.com**

Contents

1

Introduction

It is best to prove things by actual experiment; then you know; whereas if you depend on guessing and supposing and conjectures, you never get educated.

—Mark Twain

... statistics are curious things. They afford one of the few examples in which the use ... of mathematical methods tends to induce a strong emotional reaction in non-mathematical minds. This is because statisticians apply, to problems in which we are interested, a technique which we do not understand. It is exasperating, when we have studied a problem by methods that we have spent laborious years in mastering, to find our conclusions questioned, and perhaps refuted, by someone who could not have made the observations himself.

—Sir Austin Bradford Hill (1937)

1.1 A Brief History of Clinical Trials

The history of clinical trials before 1750 is easily summarized: There were no clinical trials. The basic philosophy of medicine from the time of Hippocrates to the seventeenth century was humoralistic; the accepted version of this philosophy was due to the Greek Galen (130 AD). Since he "laid down ... all that could possibly be said on medicine, he attained an authority that remained unchallenged until well into the sixteenth century. His views on cancer continued to be decisive for an even longer time" (De Moulin, 1989). Illness was caused by imbalances in blood, phlegm, black bile, and yellow bile; treatment consisted of restoring balance. Cancer was caused by a congestion of black bile; appropriate treatment was therefore rigorous purging, a strict bland diet, and, for non-occult disease, poultices and possibly surgery with evacuation of melancholic blood. No matter that the treatments didn't work—after all, preoccupation with staying alive was contemptuously worldly. (Besides, there were always the miracles of Saint Cosmas and Saint Damian if the doctors couldn't do anything.) Not until the Renaissance were the humoralistic bases questioned. Various chemical, mechanical, and electrical causes of cancer were then proposed, and treatments devised in accordance with these causes. Sadly, these treatments were just as ineffective as the theories were inaccurate (e.g.,

1

arsenic to neutralize acidic cancer juice, diets to dissolve coagulated lymph, bloodletting or shocks to remove excessive electrical irritability). It never occurred to anyone to test whether the treatments worked.

The value of numerical methods began to be appreciated in the 1800s "when in 1806, E. Duvillard in Paris, applying a primitive statistical analysis, showed the favorable effect of smallpox vaccination on the general mortality rate" (De Moulin, 1989, from Duvillard, 1806). These early methods did uncover important epidemiologic facts, but were not so useful in judging treatment effectiveness. Although patient follow-up became the norm rather than the exception, and theories became more sophisticated, typical treatment research consisted only of reports of case series. In an early example of the hazards of such research, reports of the post-operative cure of breast cancer of two Edinburgh surgeons in the 1700s (one the student of the other) were wildly divergent: One was reported as curing 4 out of 60 patients, the other as curing 76 out of 88 (De Moulin, 1989, from Monro, 1781 and Wolff, 1907). Little wonder it was nearly impossible to tell what worked and what did not.

If some of the treatments hadn't been actively harmful, perhaps it wouldn't have mattered. Despite major advances in the understanding of disease by 1900, there were still few effective treatments. "The thick textbooks of 1900 are as sweepingly accurate on diagnosis as today's, but the chapters are all tragedies because they lack a happy ending of effective treatment" (Gordon, 1993). Still, the few medical advances (mercury for syphilis, digitalis for the heart disease, iodine for goitre) and especially the advances in surgery allowed by anesthetics and antiseptics ushered in the "golden age" of Western medicine. Doctors had a priestly role as wise and trusted advisors, with warm and personal relationships with their patients (Silverman, 1992). Of course, these trusted advisors with warm personal relationships didn't experiment on their patients. Thus even though most of the principles of comparative trials had been enunciated as early as 1866 by Claude Bernard—". . . else the doctor walks at random and becomes sport of illusion" (Boissel, 1989, quoted from Bernard, 1866)—and despite the development of modern methods of experimental design in other scientific fields, clinical research remained limited.

In the middle of this century, treatment options began to catch up with biological advances: Questions abounded, and clear answers were not coming fast enough. The first randomized therapeutic clinical trial (1946–48) was the result of a pressing medical problem (tuberculosis), a severely limited supply of a new agent (streptomycin), and frustration with the uninterpretability of 100 years of uncontrolled experimentation. Sir Austin Bradford Hill made the statistical arguments for the trial: The best way to get an answer, particularly given a streptomycin supply sufficient for only 50 patients, was a strictly controlled trial (Hill, 1990). Dr. Phillip D'Arcy Hart, an expert in the treatment of tuberculosis, gave the medical arguments. "The natural course of pulmonary tuberculosis is . . . so variable and unpredictable that evidence of improvement or cure following the use of a new drug in a few cases cannot be accepted as proof of the effect of that drug. The history of chemotherapeutic trials in tuberculosis is filled with errors . . ." He went on to note that the claims made for gold treatment, which had persisted over 15 years, provided a "spectacular example" and concluded that results in the future could not be considered valid unless tested in an adequately controlled trial (Gail, 1996, quoting from Streptomycin in Tuberculosis Trials Committee of the Medical Research Council, 1948).

This first trial demonstrated convincingly that a regimen of streptomycin plus bed rest was superior to bed rest alone. Not at all bad for the first attempt: 15 years and still no answer on gold with the old observational methods, 2 years with the new methods and a clear answer on streptomycin.

The trial of streptomycin for pulmonary tuberculosis "can be seen to have ushered in a new era of medicine," and Hill generally is agreed to have done "more than any other individual to introduce and foster adoption of the properly randomized controlled trial in modern clinical research" (Silverman and Chalmers, 1991). His efforts to explain and promote good clinical research were tireless and ultimately effective, particularly after the thalidomide tragedy of the 1960s demonstrated the potential harm in *not* doing carefully controlled trials.

Controlled trials in cancer in the United States were first sponsored by the National Cancer Institute (NCI) under the leadership of Dr. Gordon Zubrod. Zubrod, profoundly influenced by the streptomycin trial, employed the new methods himself (with others) in the study of penicillin in pneumonia and introduced the methods to other early leaders in the cancer clinical trials effort (Zubrod, 1982). Upon his move to the NCI, a comparative study in childhood acute leukemia was designed. This effort expanded into two of the initial cooperative cancer clinical trials groups, the Acute Leukemia Groups A and B; Group B (which became Cancer and Leukemia Group B, or CALGB, recently merged into the Alliance for Clinical Trials in Oncology, or ACTION) had the honor of publishing the first trial (Frei et al., 1958). Zubrod was also instrumental in the formation, in 1955, of the Eastern Solid Tumor Group (now the Eastern Cooperative Oncology Group, or ECOG), which published the first randomized trial in solid tumors in the United States in 1960 (Zubrod et al., 1960).

Of course not everyone was immediately persuaded that randomized trials were the best way to conduct clinical research. Jerome Cornfield, who advised Zubrod, was a major figure in the development of biostatistical methods at the NCI and an early advocate of randomization. His response to the suggestion from a radiotherapist that patients be assigned to conventional therapy or super voltage according to hospital instead of by randomization is often quoted. The quote is a very tactfully worded suggestion that the approach would be suitable if there were no other design options. He ended with an example of a seasickness trial with treatment assigned by boat. How could the trial be interpreted if there were a great deal more turbulence and seasickness on one of the boats? The radiotherapist got the point and randomized by patient (Ederer, 1982). Cornfield is also important for his advocacy of adequate planning, attention to quality, and especially adequate sample size: ". . . clinical research . . . is littered with the wrecks of studies that are inconclusive or misleading because they were of inadequate scope" (Ederer, 1982, quoting from a memorandum to the Coronary Drug Project steering committee).

Ever since the streptomycin trial, randomized studies have been invaluable in assessing the effectiveness of new therapies. In some cases cherished beliefs have been challenged. An early example was the University Group Diabetes Project (UGDP), which contradicted the widespread view that lowering blood sugar with oral hypoglycemic drugs prolonged life in patients with diabetes. Other examples include the National Surgical Adjuvant Breast and Bowel Program (NSABP) trials of breast cancer surgery demonstrating that more is *not* better, the Cardiac Arrhythmia Suppression Trial (CAST) trial demonstrating that suppression of ventricular arrhythmia by encainide or flecainide in patients having recent myocardial infarction *increases* the death rate instead of decreasing it, and the Southwest Oncology Group (SWOG) trial in non-Hogkin's lymphoma demonstrating that new highly toxic combination chemotherapy regimens introduced in the 1980s are *not* better than the old standard combination regimen. However, cherished beliefs die hard. Results such as these met with heavy resistance despite the randomized designs (for other examples see Klimt, 1989); think how easy it would have been to dismiss the results if the designs had been inherently biased. Positive results are happier examples of the importance of clinical trials: The Diabetic Retinopathy Trial demonstrating dramatically reduced visual loss due to photocoagulation therapy, trials establishing the effectiveness of therapy in improving survival in patients with Wilms' tumor and other childhood cancers, beta blockers prolonging life after myocardial infarction, chemo-radiotherapy substantially improving survival in nasopharyngeal and gastric cancers.

Randomized trials cannot answer every treatment question. Randomization is not feasible in every setting, costs may be prohibitive, and political realities may interfere. Since only a limited number of trials can be done, some questions have to be addressed in other ways. However, controlled trials are by far the best method available for addressing difficult and controversial questions in a way that minimizes distrust of the results. Consider the 1954 Salk Vaccine trial for which at the beginning "the most urgent business was to . . . turn the focus away from professional rivalries, power struggles, and theoretical disputes and back to the neglected question of whether or not Salk's vaccine worked." Thomas Francis, Jr., was given the job of evaluating the vaccine because "everybody knew that when Tommy Francis talked about working up to a standard, it was one of unimpeachable thoroughness; even the most dedicated opponent to the new vaccine could never say a trial supervised by Francis was political, biased, or incomplete" (Smith, 1990). His two nonnegotiable demands before agreeing to take on the job were that the vaccine proponents would not design the trial and would have no access to the results while the trial was ongoing, and that the trial would have a randomized double blind design instead of an "observed-control" design, in which second graders would have gotten the vaccine and would have been compared to unvaccinated first and third graders (Smith, 1992, quotes from Smith, 1990). The results of this "textbook model of elegant clinical testing" were unquestionable. Francis's announcement that "the new vaccine was safe, effective, and potent ... was a landmark in 20th century history, one of the few events that burned itself into the public consciousness because the news was good" (Smith, 1992). Unimpeachable thoroughness, nonpolitical, unbiased, complete, independent, properly designed—Francis set a very high standard indeed, and one to which all of us involved in clinical research should aspire.

1.2 The Southwest Oncology Group (SWOG)

There are now dozens of national and international consortia of institutions and investigators organized for the purpose of improving the survival of cancer patients through clinical research. Our own experience is with the Southwest Oncology Group, now known simply as SWOG, which began in 1956 in the United States as the (pediatric) Southwest Cancer Chemotherapy Study Group under the direction of Dr. Grant Taylor at the M.D. Anderson Cancer Center in Houston, Texas. In 1958, membership was extended to include investigators evaluating adult malignancies, and in the early 1960s a Solid Tumor Committee was established. Since then the pediatric part of the Group was split off (to become the Pediatric Oncology Group, now part of the Children's Oncology Group), the name was changed to the Southwest Oncology Group (SWOG), and the Group has expanded to include specialists in all modalities of cancer therapy and institutions in all regions of the country. Most of the studies done by the Group are designed to assess whether a regimen merits further study (Phase II), or to compare two or more regimens (Phase III). Studies in cancer control research (prevention, symptom control and quality of life, survivorship) are also carried out. Currently the Group is led by the Group Chair, Dr. Laurence Baker (University of Michigan, Ann Arbor) and the Group Statistician, Dr. John Crowley (Cancer Research and Biostatistics and Fred Hutchinson Cancer Research Center, Seattle).

The structure of SWOG is typical of cooperative groups and includes the group chair's office (administration, grants management, industry contracts, legal matters), the operations office (protocol development, meeting planning, regulatory requirements, audits); the statistical center (study development, data base management, network services, computer applications, study quality control, statistical analysis and statistical research); disease committees (breast cancer, gastrointestinal cancer, genitourinary cancer, leukemia, lung cancer, lymphoma, melanoma, myeloma); discipline committees (such as radiotherapy, surgery, nursing and clinical research associates); cancer control and prevention committees (prevention, molecular epidemiology, outcomes and comparative effectiveness, survivorship, and symptom control and quality of life); and all of the participating institutions that enter patients on trials. Group trials and related scientific investigations are proposed and developed within the disease committees under the leadership of the disease committee chairs. Committee leadership is also provided by the disease committee statistician, who is responsible for reviewing, designing, monitoring and analyzing all studies done in the committee. Each study developed has a clinician assigned (the "study coordinator") to lead the development effort, to evaluate the data after the study is open, and to be the primary author on the manuscript when the study is complete. Each study also has a "protocol coordinator" assigned from the operations office, who coordinates the production and review of the study protocol, and a "data coordinator" from the statistical center who does most of the necessary setup work for opening a study and reviews and evaluates all of the study data. Participating physicians and clinical research associates at Group institutions are responsible for submitting protocols to their Institutional Review Board, identifying patients suitable for studies, obtaining informed consent, ensuring study participants are treated and followed according to protocol, and for correctly submitting all required data.

The Group typically has 80–100 actively accruing studies at any one time and 400 closed studies in active follow-up. Over 4000 physicians from more than 400 institutions participate. Since the Group began, over 150,000 patients have been registered to its studies, and over 2,000 abstracts and manuscripts have been published. The Group's extensive clinical trials experience provides the context and many of the examples for this book.

1.3 The Reason for This Book

Our motivations for writing this book are captured by the introductory quotes. Among the four of us we have devoted over 100 years to clinical trials research. As suggested by the first quote, we want to know whether treatments work or not. Furthermore, we want the methods we use to find out whether treatments work to be unimpeachable. Unfortunately, as suggested by the second quote, as statisticians we too often find our motives and methods misunderstood or questioned—and at times actively resented. With this book, it is our hope to improve the mutual understanding by clinicians and statisticians of the principles of cancer clinical trials. Although many of the examples we use are specific to SWOG, the issues and principles discussed are important in cancer clinical trials more generally, and indeed in any clinical trials setting.

2

Statistical Concepts

To understand God's thoughts we must study statistics, for these are the measure of His purpose.

—Florence Nightingale

2.1 Introduction

A collaborative team that includes both clinicians and statisticians is crucial to the successful conduct of a clinical trial. Although the statistical study design and analyses are mainly the responsibility of the statistician, an understanding of the basic statistical principles is vital for the clinicians involved with the study. The main goal of this chapter is to present statistical concepts that are of particular application to cancer clinical trials.

The objectives of the trial, the key types of data that are collected to meet these objectives, and the types of analyses to be performed are in large part determined by the type of study being undertaken. Phase II trials (discussed in Chapter 5) are small studies early in the development of a regimen that typically focus on toxicity and short-term efficacy data, while Phase III trials (discussed in Chapter 6) are large comparative studies that most frequently assess survival and progression-free survival. We will introduce statistical concepts within the context of each of these types of studies. Phase I trials (discussed in Chapter 4) are a third type of clinical trial which involve a much smaller number of patients, and as such are less suited for use in illustrating basic statistical principles.

First, however, there are some general characteristics of data from clinical trials that do not depend on the type of study. Outcome measures can be classified as being either (1) categorical (qualitative) or (2) measurement (quantitative).

1. Categorical data—outcomes that can be classified according to one of several mutually exclusive categories based on a predetermined set of criteria. For example, standard criteria for solid tumor response (RECIST 1.1, Eisenhauer et al., 2009) categorize patients as achieving

either a CR (complete response) if there is normalization of malignant nodes and disappearance of all other disease; a PR (partial response) if the sum of the diameters of target measurable lesions (shortest diameter for nodes, longest for other lesions) reduces by 30% or more from baseline; INC (increasing) if the diameters increase by 20% or more, or if new sites of tumor are noted; and STA (stable) if none of the above occur. Thus, in this case, patient response can be described by one of four categories, which are then often dichotomized into two categories for analysis (CR + PR versus others; INC versus others).

2. Measured data—outcomes that are measured quantities. For example, concentrations of CA-125, a tumor antigen, are routinely collected in trials of ovarian cancer. Levels of this antigen range in value from 0 to over 10,000. In this case, the data measure a quantity that takes on many possible values. An important special case of quantitative data is time to event data, such as survival time, a measurement in units of time from entry on a study until death. What distinguishes this outcome, and its analysis, from other quantitative data is the frequent presence of what statisticians call censoring. In a typical clinical trial, not all patients have died by the time the study is completed and analyses are performed. For patients still alive, we know that they have lived at least as long as the time from the patient's entry on the study to the time of the analysis, but we don't know the actual death time. Special statistical techniques have been developed to incorporate these right censored observations into the analysis.

Three other general concepts we introduce in this section are *probability, statistic,* and *distribution.* The *probability* of an outcome is how often that outcome occurs in relation to all possible outcomes. For instance, the set of all possible outcomes for a flip of a coin is $\{H, T\}$. The probability of outcome T (tails) is $1/2$ if the coin is fair. If the coin is unfair (or biased) and the outcome H (heads) is twice as likely as T, the set of all possible outcomes remains $\{H, T\}$ but the probability of T is now $1/3$. If the coin is flipped twice, the set of possible outcomes is $\{HH, HT, TH, TT\}$. Note that there are two events that yield exactly one tail in two flips, since the tail can be the outcome of either the first or the second flip. With the fair coin the probability of TT is $1/2 \times 1/2 = 1/4$; with the biased coin it is $1/3 \times 1/3 = 1/9$. The probability of exactly one tail is $(1/2 \times 1/2) + (1/2 \times 1/2) = 1/2$ or $(1/3 \times 2/3) + (2/3 \times 1/3) = 4/9$ for the fair and biased coin, respectively. Multiplying the probabilities on each flip to arrive at a probability for the outcomes of events such as TT or HT is justified by an assumption of independence of coin flips, i.e., that the probability of tails on the second flip is unaffected by the outcome of the first flip.

Most commonly used statistical procedures require this independence assumption. What this means is that the value of one observation provides no information about the value of any other. In particular, two measures from the same patient can not be treated as if they were from two separate (independent) patients. This is because two measurements on the same patient tend to be more alike than two measurements from two different people. Treating multiple observations (such as results from multiple biopsy specimens as to the presence of the multi-drug resistance gene, or MDR) as independent is a common pitfall that should be avoided. For instance, if half of all patients have MDR positive tumors, but within a patient multiple biopsy results are nearly always the same, then about 3/6 patients would be expected to have MDR positive tumors if all 6 biopsies were from different patients, while either 0/6 or 6/6 biopsies would be expected to be positive if all 6 were from the same patient.

The outcome "number of MDR positive tumors out of N tumors" is an example of a *statistic*, that is, a summary of results from N separate tumors. In general, a statistic is any summary from a set of data points. For example, in the case of measured data such as CA-125, one could summarize the measures from a group of patients using descriptive statistics such as a mean or a median. The statistics chosen to summarize a data set will depend on the type of data collected and the intended use of the information. Some statistics are merely descriptive; others, called test statistics, are used to test hypotheses after the data from an experiment are collected.

A *distribution* characterizes the probabilities of all possible outcomes of an event or all possible values of a statistic. For a single flip of a fair coin the distribution is

$$\text{outcome} \quad H \quad T$$
$$\text{probability} \quad 1/2 \quad 1/2\,'$$

while for the biased coin it is

$$\text{outcome} \quad H \quad T$$
$$\text{probability} \quad 2/3 \quad 1/3\,.$$

When a coin is flipped multiple times, a statistic often used to summarize the outcome is the number of tails observed. The distribution of this statistic is the *binomial* distribution, the most important distribution for categorical data. The distribution from an experiment of flipping a coin N times is characterized by giving the probability that the number of tails is equal to k, for every k from 0 to N. If the probability of a tail on one flip is p, and the flips are independent, the probability of any sequence of flips yielding exactly k tails (and thus $N - k$ heads) is $p^k(1 - p)^{N-k}$. The rest of the exercise is to figure out how many sequences of heads and tails have exactly k tails, and add those up. For $N = 2$ and $k = 1$, we saw above that there were two such sequences, HT and TH. In general, the answer is given by the formula $\binom{N}{k} = \frac{N!}{k!(N-k)!}$, where $\binom{N}{k}$ is read "N choose k" and N! is N "factorial," which is simply $N \times (N-1) \times \cdots \times 2 \times 1$. Thus the probability of exactly three tails in six flips of a fair coin is $\binom{6}{3}(1/2)^3(1 - 1/2)^{6-3} = \frac{6!}{3!3!}(1/2)^6 = 20/64 = 5/16 = 0.3125$. The entire binomial distribution for $N = 6$, and $p = 1/2$ or $1/3$ is given in Figure 2.1 (part (a) for $p = \frac{1}{2}$; part (b) for $p = \frac{1}{3}$).

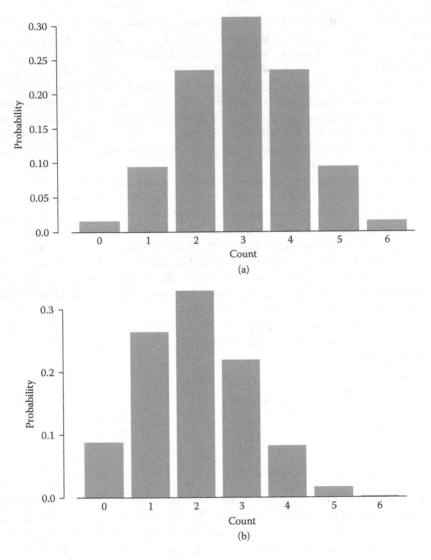

FIGURE 2.1
The binomial distribution for $N = 6$ and (a) $p = \frac{1}{2}$, (b) $p = \frac{1}{3}$.

Binomial distributions apply in countless settings other than coin flips; the one of most interest to us in this book is tumor response (the number of responses in N patients taking the place of the number of tails in N flips). In the MDR example above, the binomial distribution applies only to the case where all biopsies are from different patients, since independence is a requirement for the distribution. The probability of exactly three MDR positive patients out of six, if the probability is 1/2 for an individual patient, is 0.3125; if all six biopsies are from the same patient this probability is close to 0. Applying the binomial distribution to the second case is clearly inappropriate.

When outcomes are categorical, the distribution can be shown in a simple table or graph, as above. When outcomes are measured, the distribution can't be described in a table. Instead, cumulative probabilities are described by a function $F(t)$. For time to death, for example, $F(t)$ means the probability of dying before time t. The derivative of $F(t)$, denoted $f(t)$ and often called the density, can be thought of loosely as the probability of dying at t (in a sense made precise by the calculus). We also often talk more optimistically of the survival curve $S(t) = 1 - F(t)$, the probability of surviving at least to time t. Note that $S(0) = 1$ and $S(t)$ decreases towards 0 as t gets large. The *median* survival time, the time past which one half of the patients are expected to live, is that time m for which $S(m) = 0.5$.

Yet another quantity of interest is the *hazard function* or *hazard rate*, often denoted $\lambda(t)$. This function can be thought of loosely as the probability of death at time t given that the patient is alive just before time t: the instantaneous rate of failure. In terms of the other quantities we have described, the hazard function is given by $\lambda(t) = f(t)/S(t)$. Depending upon the type of disease, the hazard rate as a function of time can take on a variety of forms. For example, in a study involving surgery, a patient's risk of dying may be highest during the post operative period, then decrease for a period of time. A rising hazard function is characteristic of normal mortality as one ages. In an advanced disease trial, the risk of dying may be relatively constant over the time of follow-up. These three types of hazard functions are given in Figure 2.2a, with the corresponding survival curves in Figure 2.2b.

The constant hazard case with $\lambda(t) = \lambda$ gives rise to what is called the exponential distribution, for which the survival curve is given by

$$S(t) = \exp(-\lambda t),$$

where exp is the exponential function. Under the assumption of exponential survival, the median survival m is

$$m = -\ln(0.5)/\lambda,$$

where ln is the natural logarithm. From this relationship it is easy to note that the ratio of hypothesized median survival times for two treatment arms is equal to the inverse of the ratio of the hypothesized hazards. Figure 2.3 shows the hazard function, survival curve, and median survival for an exponential distribution. Although the assumption of a constant hazard rate may not be correct in practice, it can be used to provide reasonable sample size estimates for designing clinical trials (see Chapter 6).

The most common quantitative distribution is the "normal" or "Gaussian" distribution, or "bell-shaped curve." The standard normal density $f(x)$, presented in Figure 2.4, is a symmetric curve about the mean value 0. The probability of an outcome being less than x is $F(x)$, the area under the density up to x. The area under the whole curve has the value 1. The probability that an observation with this standard normal distribution is negative (zero or smaller) is $1/2$, the area under the curve to the left of 0 ($F(0) = 0.5$). The probability

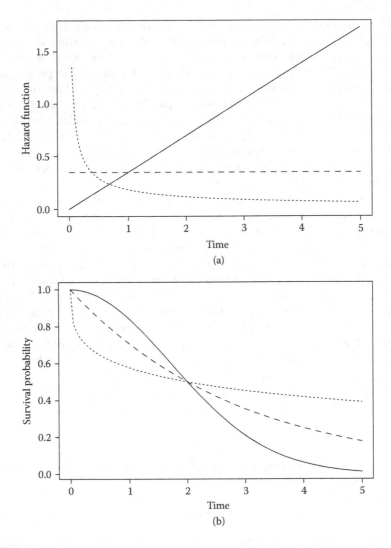

FIGURE 2.2
(a) Increasing (solid line), decreasing (dotted line), and constant (dashed line) hazard functions;
(b) corresponding survival curves.

that an observation is greater than 1.645 is 0.05, and the probability that an observation is between -1.96 and 1.96 is 0.95. The beauty of the normal distribution is that as sample sizes get large many common statistics that start out as non-normal attain an approximately normal distribution (or a distribution related to the normal, such as the χ^2 discussed in Section 2.3.1). This fact is embodied mathematically in what is known as the Central Limit Theorem. For instance, the probability of k or fewer tails in N coin flips can be found (approximately) from the normal distribution. This is useful in the development of statistical tests, and in the estimation of sample sizes (see Section 2.5).

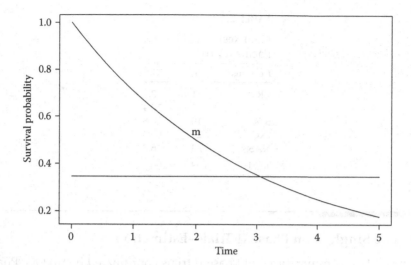

FIGURE 2.3
Hazard function (horizontal line), survival curve, and median survival (m) for an exponential distribution.

The remainder of this chapter has been designed to present the key statistical concepts related to cancer clinical trials. For the most part, formulas will only be presented to provide insight into the use of certain statistical tests and procedures; it is far more important to understand *why* certain statistical techniques are used, rather than *how* to use them. We will begin with examples that will be used to illustrate the key concepts.

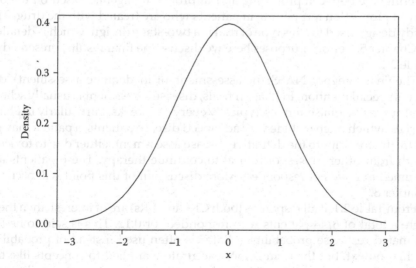

FIGURE 2.4
The standard normal density curve.

TABLE 2.1

Final Results of Phase II
Paclitaxel Trial

Response	N	%
CR	1	2.1
PR	5	10.4
STA	10	20.8
INC	29	60.4
NASS	3	6.3
Total	48	100

2.2 The Single-Arm Phase II Trial—Estimation

There are two common types of Phase II trials coordinated by SWOG. Phase II trials of Investigational New Drugs (INDs) are performed in order to assess whether a new drug shows some promise of activity for a particular disease type. Phase II pilot studies are usually done to assess activity and feasibility of previously tested treatments, either using a new treatment schedule, and/or using the drug in combination with other agents or modalities. In either case, care must be taken to explicitly define what is meant by "show some activity," "assess activity," or "evaluate feasibility."

SWOG S9134 (Balcerzak et al., 1995) was a Phase II IND trial that studied whether paclitaxel had any effectiveness in shrinking tumors of patients with soft tissue sarcomas. Typically, the formal goal of a Phase II IND trial is to discriminate between promising and unpromising agents, based on the observed proportion responding in patients who are treated with the drug. The study design used for this type of trial is a two-stage design, which is detailed in Chapter 5. For our purposes here we discuss the final results, presented in Table 2.1.

The final category, NASS, (no assessment, or inadequate assessment), deserves special mention. In Phase II trials, disease assessment is usually scheduled at specific time intervals, typically every 4–8 weeks. Particularly in Phase II trials, which often include very advanced disease patients, a patient may go off treatment prior to the definitive disease assessment, either due to toxicity, death from other causes, or refusal to continue therapy. These patients are assumed to have not responded. More discussion of this point will occur in Chapter 8.

From Table 2.1, if all responses (both CRs and PRs) are of interest, then there were a total of 6/48 patients who responded, or 0.12. This is said to be the estimated response probability. ("Rate" is often used instead of probability in this context, but the term is more accurately applied to concepts like the hazard.) The word "estimate" is used since this is not a true probability, but an approximation calculated from a sample of 48 individuals who were recruited for this trial. If the same trial were repeated in 48 different individuals, one would not expect that the estimated response probability for this second group of patients would be exactly 0.12, but might be smaller, or larger. If repeated trials were done, there would be a distribution of estimates of the response probability. This is due to the fact that each individual trial is made up of a sample of individuals from a larger population. In this example the larger population consists of all patients with soft tissue sarcoma who would satisfy the eligibility criteria of the study. If we could treat the entire population of patients with paclitaxel, we would know the true response probability. What we hope, instead, is to use our sample of patients to get a reasonable estimate of the true probability, and to distinguish unpromising agents (with low true response probabilities) from promising ones. Symbolically, we denote the true response probability in the population by p, and denote the estimate of p from the sample of patients in the trial by $\widehat{p}$ (here 0.12).

Accompanying this idea of an estimate of a true, but unknown, response probability is the notion of precision, or variability of our estimate. Because each estimate from a sample of individuals is not always going to produce a value that is exactly the same as the true response probability, we wish to have some assessment of how close our estimate is to the truth. This assessment depends, in large measure, on how many patients were studied. To understand this, consider the clinical trial of size 1. With one patient, an estimated response probability of either 0 or 1 are the only values that can be obtained. Yet no one would feel comfortable using that estimate as being reflective of the population. As the sample size increases, we begin to feel more confident that the resulting estimate comes close to measuring the true response probability. Thus, in a series of studies of 100 patients each, we would expect to see more precise estimates (less variability) than we would in a series of studies based on 48 patients. To illustrate this, consider Figure 2.5. These graphs are called histograms, and are a display of the frequency of values from a collection of data. Figure 2.5a displays the estimates of the response probabilities from a series of 100 studies, all based on 40 patients, while Figure 2.5b graphs the same results based on samples of size 100. In each case, the data are generated by the computer assuming the same true response probability $p = 0.20$. It can be seen that the results based on trials of size 100 are more closely clustered around the value $p = 0.20$ than are the results based on a sample of size 40. Also notice that the shape of the distribution for trials of size 100 is closer to that of the normal distribution in Figure 2.4 than is the shape for trials of size 40.

The notion of precision of an estimate is often expressed as an interval of values that we could reasonably expect will include the true probability. This range of values is called a confidence interval. In the above paclitaxel example, the 95% confidence interval for the response probability is 0.047 to 0.253. This interval was obtained from some tables specifically designed for the binomial distribution (Diem and Lentner, 1970). Good approximations to this exact interval are possible when the sample size is large using the normal distribution, as explained in Section 2.1. The way we interpret this interval is to say that we are 95% confident that the true response probability

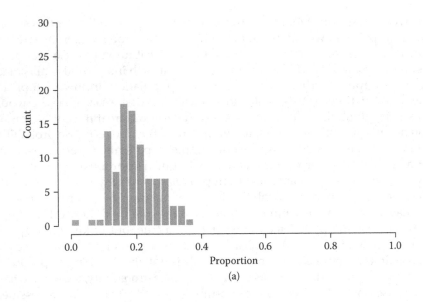

(a)

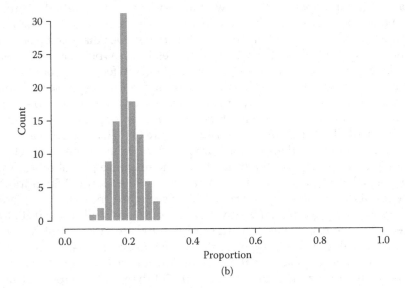

(b)

FIGURE 2.5
Histogram of estimated response probabilities from a series of 100 studies, each with (a) 40 patients, (b) 100 patients.

(in the population) is somewhere between 0.047 and 0.253, in the sense that in a series of similar trials the 95% confidence interval will contain the true population probability 95% of the time. Investigators may choose other levels of confidence for the interval, depending on how sure they want to be that the true value is in the interval. A 90% confidence interval may be sufficient

TABLE 2.2

Dependence of Confidence
Interval Width on Sample
Size when $\hat{p} = 0.2$

N	Confidence Interval
20	(0.06, 0.44)
40	(0.09, 0.36)
60	(0.11, 0.32)
80	(0.12, 0.30)

for a Phase II trial, while 99% may be desirable when it is important to be conservative in drawing conclusions.

Suppose now that the researcher wishes to base a decision on whether to pursue treatment of soft tissue sarcoma with paclitaxel on the results of this Phase II trial. The results of this trial, with $\hat{p} = 0.12$, are consistent with a true response probability that is very low, or with an agent of modest activity. If the researcher were interested in finding a drug that was believed to have at least a 0.30 response probability, then this trial would lead the researcher to conclude that paclitaxel was not sufficiently active, and to pursue other therapies.

With a small sample size, the width of the confidence interval will be wide, implying that there is a large range of possible values for the true response probability; if the sample size is large, the corresponding confidence interval is much narrower. Table 2.2 gives the width of the confidence intervals obtained from four trials of sample sizes 20, 40, 60, and 80, all yielding the same response estimate of 0.20. Thus the notion of a confidence interval provides a measure of the precision of the estimate.

We have already mentioned the concept of a sample of patients from some larger population. A key aspect of any study is the reliability with which we may generalize the results we observe in our sample to the target population of interest. We discussed the impact of the size of our sample on our ability to draw reliable conclusions. Of equal importance is the similarity of our sample to the population to which we wish to apply the results of the study. For example, in the soft tissue sarcoma trial, we may wish to test paclitaxel for use in all patients with poor prognosis soft tissue sarcoma. However, if only patients with uterine leiomyosarcoma are included in the Phase II trial, then the resulting response probability may underestimate that which would have been seen in patients with other histologic types, since uterine leiomyosarcomas are traditionally unresponsive to chemotherapy. This lack of similarity in the sample and target population results in estimates that are biased; that is, they yield estimates that are not reflective of the population of interest. Care must be taken in defining eligibility criteria and in selecting patients in order to ensure that the population sampled is representative of the population to which generalizations are to be made.

2.3   The Randomized Phase III Trial—Hypothesis Testing

The goal of the Phase III trial is to compare treatment regimens. Early medicine based decisions on anecdotal reports of therapeutic successes, or, more recently, on case series or prospective but nonrandomized trials. In these studies, groups of patients were given the therapy of interest. Results were then compared to historical knowledge or reports of patient experience with other treatments (see Chapter 1). Because of the huge potential for differences in the patient populations in these trials, biases are impossible to completely remove, making decisions based on nonrandomized trials subject to question. Since one of the major sources of bias is the unmeasurable process by which physicians and patients make treatment decisions, it is widely acknowledged that the most appropriate way to compare treatments is through a randomized clinical trial. Patients who satisfy the eligibility criteria of the trial are randomly assigned to treatment. This randomization guarantees that there is no systematic selection bias in treatment allocation. Techniques for randomization are discussed in Chapter 6. Examples of historical controls are presented in Chapter 9.

The primary objective for a Phase III trial in cancer is generally to compare survival (or disease-free or progression-free survival) among the treatment regimens. However, dichotomized categorical outcomes such as response are also often compared, and for ease of exposition we start with this dichotomous case.

2.3.1   Response as the Outcome

SWOG S8412 (Alberts et al., 1992) was a study of the use of cyclophosphamide and either carboplatin or cisplatin in patients with Stage III or Stage IV ovarian cancer. One of the objectives (though not the primary one) was to compare the study arms with respect to response to chemotherapy in patients with measurable disease. Patients were randomized to receive either carboplatin and cyclophosphamide or cisplatin and cyclophosphamide, and were followed for survival and response. Of 291 eligible patients, 124 had measurable disease. We can record the response results of the trial in Table 2.3, called a 2×2 contingency table:

TABLE 2.3

Responses to Treatment for Ovarian Cancer

	Response	No Response	Totals	Response Estimate
Arm A	31	29	60	0.52
Arm B	39	25	64	0.61
Totals	70	54	124	0.565

Note that for each treatment, we can estimate the response probability as we did for the Phase II trial above. Thus, the estimated response probability for the cisplatin arm (denoted arm A) is $\hat{p}_A = 31/60 = 0.52$ and for the carboplatin arm (arm B) it is $\hat{p}_B = 39/64 = 0.61$. Each estimate is based on the number of patients in the respective groups.

Because our goal here is to compare treatments, the question of interest is whether the response probability for patients receiving cisplatin differs from that for patients receiving carboplatin. We can phrase this as a hypothesis. The null hypothesis (denoted by H_0) for this illustration is that $p_A = p_B$, or in statistical shorthand, $H_0 : p_A = p_B$.

The *alternative hypothesis,* or H_1, which most often is what we are interested in establishing, could take one of two basic forms. If Treatment A is a more toxic or costly new regimen and Treatment B is a standard, the alternative hypothesis might be that the new regimen is better than the old. In statistical terms, this is written as $H_1 : p_A > p_B$. We will stay with the status quo (Treatment B) unless the new regimen proves to be better (we are not really interested in proving whether the new regimen is worse). This is known as a *one-sided* test. If Treatment A and Treatment B are two competing standards, we might be interested in seeing if one of the two is better. This *two-sided* alternative is denoted $H_1 : p_A \neq p_B$.

If the null hypothesis is true, then we would expect that the difference in our estimated probabilities, $\hat{p}_A - \hat{p}_B$, should be close to zero, while if there were really a difference between the two true probabilities, we would expect the difference in the estimated probabilities to be much different from zero. In a manner similar to what we did for the Phase II trial, we can create a confidence interval for the difference between the two probabilities. In this case, the 95% confidence interval (based on the approximation using the normal distribution) is $(-0.26, 0.08)$. Because this interval contains zero, it is consistent with the hypothesis that the difference is zero; that is, that the true probabilities p_A and p_B are the same. If the interval did not include 0, the data would be more consistent with the hypothesis that the difference is nonzero.

There is another way to test the hypothesis that the two probabilities are equal. Based on the data we observe, we would like a formal way of deciding when the null hypothesis is false (and not be wrong very often). That is, are the true response probabilities p_A and p_B really different, based on estimates of 0.52 and 0.61 with these sample sizes? A statistical test of this hypothesis can be formulated in the following way. From Table 2.3, we see that overall, $70/124 = 0.565$ of the patients responded to chemotherapy. If there were no differences in the two regimens, we would expect about 0.565 of the patients receiving cisplatin to respond (or $0.565 \times 60 = 33.87 \approx 34$ patients), and about 0.435 of them (26) to fail to respond. Similarly, we would expect about 36 of the patients receiving carboplatin to respond, and 28 to fail to respond. How different is what we observe from what we would expect? A number used to summarize the discrepancy between the observed and expected values under the null hypothesis is called the χ^2 (Chi-squared). It is computed as $\chi^2 = \sum [(observed–expected)^2/expected]$, where the summation means sum

TABLE 2.4

Notation Used in χ^2 Test of 2×2 Contingency Table

	Response	No Response	Totals
Arm A	r_A	$n_A - r_A$	n_A
Arm B	r_B	$n_B - r_B$	n_B
Totals	r	$n - r$	n

over the four entries in the 2×2 table. The χ^2 is an example of a test statistic. It is appropriate when the data are categorical; that is, each observation can be classified, as in this example, according to characteristics such as treatment arm and response. A second requirement for the χ^2 test (and most commonly used statistical tests) is independence of observations.

If there were perfect agreement between the observed and expected values, the χ^2 value would be zero. The greater the discrepancy in the observed and expected values, the greater the value of the χ^2. In this case, we would have

$$(31 - 33.87)^2/33.87 + (29 - 26.13)^2/26.13 + (39 - 36.13)^2/36.13$$
$$+ (25 - 27.87)^2/27.87 = 1.08$$

A simpler but algebraically equivalent formula uses just one cell of the 2×2 table (any one) and the marginal totals. The notation is given in Table 2.4. Using the number of responses on arm A for specificity, the formula is $(r_A - n_A r/n)^2/[n_A n_B r(n - r)/n^3]$. Note that the numerator is still of the form $(observed-expected)^2$. With the data in Table 2.3, this is $124^3(31 - 60 \times 70/124)^2/60 \times 64 \times 70 \times 54 = 1.08$. In some circumstances this formula is modified slightly to $(r_A - n_A r/n)^2/[n_A n_B r(n - r)/n^2(n - 1)]$, as in the logrank test defined in Section 2.3.2; in other cases a modification known as the continuity-corrected χ^2 is used.

If we were to perform the same clinical trial again in 124 different patients, we would get a different value for the χ^2 test, since we would expect the new sample of patients to have a somewhat different set of responses. Thus, the statistic can take on a variety of values, characterized by a density as in Figure 2.6. When the null hypothesis is true, we can compute the probability that the χ^2 statistic exceeds certain values by looking at the appropriate area under the curve in Figure 2.6, or using a table of the χ^2 distribution. From Figure 2.6, we would find that the probability of observing a value of 1.08 or greater is very common (it can happen about 30% of the time) under the assumption that the two probabilities are equal (the null hypothesis is true). Thus, we would reason that there is not sufficient evidence to conclude that the drug regimens are different.

Use of the χ^2 distribution is actually an approximation which is reasonably accurate unless sample sizes are small. When sample sizes are small, the exact solution is known as Fisher's exact test. The appropriateness of the χ^2 distribution for larger sample sizes is a useful consequence of the Central Limit Theorem discussed in Section 2.1. In fact, distributions of many statistical tests can be approximated by a standard normal or a χ^2 distribution.

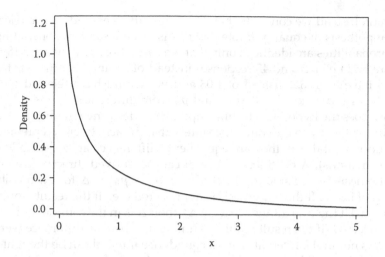

FIGURE 2.6
The chi-squared distribution (with 1 degree of freedom).

We are now ready for a more formal introduction to the idea of hypothesis testing. In the above clinical trial we wished to test $H_0 : p_A = p_B$. We performed the trial, and based on the data, made a decision about the populations. The consequences of this decision relative to the true values of p_A and p_B are summarized below:

		Truth	
		$p_A = p_B$	$p_A \neq p_B$
	Accept H_0	Correct	Type II error
Decision			
	Reject H_0	Type I error	Correct

The Type I error probability, or α, or significance level, is the probability that we conclude in our trial that the two treatments are different, even though they really aren't (false positive). The acceptable Type I error rate is decided in the planning stages of the trial. The most common significance level for testing is 0.05. In our example, if we wish to test whether the treatments are different using a 0.05 significance level, we first consider the distribution of our χ^2 statistic when there are no true differences (under the null hypothesis). How large does the χ^2 have to be before we decide that the treatments are different? As just explained, the probability under the null hypothesis that a χ^2 statistic is greater than any particular value x can be found from Figure 2.6 as the area under the curve for values of x and above, or from published tables. For $x = 3.84$ the area is 0.05. Thus if we conclude that p_A and p_B are different only when the χ^2 statistic is greater than 3.84, we know we will only be making a Type I error 5% of the time. Next we consider the observed value of our statistic, 1.08. Since it is less than 3.84, we do not conclude that p_A and p_B are different. Instead we conclude that there is insufficient evidence to reject the null hypothesis of equality. (Note that this is not the same as concluding the two probabilities are identical, only that we cannot prove they are different.) If there had been 27 and 43 responses instead of 31 and 39, our test statistic would have been 6.2 instead of 1.08 and we would have rejected the null hypothesis and concluded that p_A and p_B were different.

How does the hypothesis testing approach to deciding whether p_A and p_B are different relate to the confidence interval approach described previously? In a fundamental way they are equivalent (differences arise due to various approximations). A confidence interval can be derived directly from a test of hypothesis by considering tests of $H : p_A - p_B = \Delta$ for all possible Δ instead of just 0. If the hypothesis is not rejected (i.e., if the result would not be unusual if the true difference were Δ), then Δ is in the confidence interval; if it is rejected (if the result would be unusual if the true difference were Δ), then Δ is not in the interval. Thus a confidence interval can be thought of as the set of all possible values for which a test of hypothesis does not reject the null hypothesis. In particular, if 0 is in the confidence interval for $p_A - p_B$, the null hypothesis of no difference is not rejected; if 0 is not in the interval, the null hypothesis is rejected.

A concept related to the significance level α of a test is the p-value, the probability under the null hypothesis of a result equal to or more extreme than the one we observed. The p-value for our example is the probability of obtaining a statistic with the value 1.08 or greater, which is 0.3. If the statistic had been 6.63, the p-value would have been 0.013. By definition the smaller the p-value the less likely the observed result under the null hypothesis. When there is little chance of having obtained an observed result under the null hypothesis, we conclude that the null hypothesis is not true. Note the correspondence between p-values and the observed value of the test statistic. The rule for rejecting the null hypothesis can be stated either as "reject if the test statistic is greater than 3.84" or "reject if the p-value is less than 0.05."

As noted above, distributions of many test statistics can be approximated by the normal distribution or the χ^2 distribution, which is related to the normal distribution. Thus, p-values from many statistical tests can be approximated by finding the area to the right of an observed value using either the standard normal curve or the χ^2 distribution. Tables of the normal and χ^2 distribution can be found in any standard statistical text, for example Rosner (1986).

For a normal distribution the area to the right of the observed value is the p-value corresponding to a one-sided test. One-sided tests are used when only a specified direction (e.g., $A > B$) is of interest. In this case $A < B$ or $A = B$ lead to the same conclusion (B is the preferred treatment), so we have a Type I error only if we erroneously conclude that $A > B$. For a two-sided test differences in both directions are of interest, so we make a Type I error if we conclude either $A > B$ or $B > A$ when there is no difference. The p-value is this case is twice the area to the right of the observed value, to allow for a difference of the same or greater magnitude in either direction. For instance, the area under the normal curve above 1.96 is 0.025, so if a test statistic is equal to 1.96 the p-value for a one-sided test would be 0.025 while the p-value for a two-sided test would be 0.05. The χ^2 test statistic is inherently two-sided due to the squaring of the differences, which eliminates the indication of direction. Note that 1.96^2 is 3.84, the value for which the p-value of a χ^2 statistic would be 0.05. The decision of whether to perform a one-sided or two-sided test depends upon the goals of the study and should be specified during study development (see Section 8.3.3).

While we can predetermine the significance level of a test of hypothesis directly, the probability β of a Type II error is dependent upon several things: (1) sample size; (2) the true difference between p_A and p_B; and (3) the significance level of the test. If the true difference is very large (for example p_A near 1 and p_B near 0), we would expect that it would be relatively easy to determine that a difference in probabilities exists, even with a small sample size. However, if p_A and p_B are very close, though not equal, it might take a very large number of patients to detect this difference with near certainty. Thus, a trial which failed to detect a difference, but which was based on a small sample size, does not prove $p_A = p_B$, and should be reported with caution (since if the true difference is modest, a Type II error or false negative result is likely).

The power of a test for a particular alternative hypothesis is defined to be $1 - \beta$, i.e., the probability of detecting a difference that is really there. Ideally, we would always like to have a large enough sample size to ensure high power for differences that are realistic and clinically meaningful. In designing clinical studies, it is important for the clinician and statistician to discuss the magnitudes of the clinical differences that would be meaningful to detect, in order to design a study with small enough error rates to make the conclusions from the results credible.

2.3.2 Survival as the Outcome

In most Phase III cancer clinical trials, the primary outcome is patient survival. Patients are randomized to two (or more) groups, and followed until death. In a typical Phase III trial, there is an accrual period (often several years long), and then some additional follow-up time prior to analysis of the data. At the time of the final analysis, some patients will have died, while some patients will remain alive. For those patients who remain alive, the total time of observation will vary, depending upon when in the accrual period they were registered to the trial. The actual survival time for these patients is unknown, but we do know that they have survived at least from registration until the date of their last known contact. This represents a minimum survival time. Data of this type are described as being subject to censoring. We illustrate statistical issues related to censored data using the survival times from Table 2.5, which represent the ordered survival times for the patients on an imaginary trial. Times with a + next to them represent censored observations.

Given data of this type, we frequently wish to calculate some statistic which summarizes patient survival experience. It is not uncommon to see

TABLE 2.5

Ordered Survival Times (in Months) on an Imaginary Trial

Time (months)
1
2
4+
6
6
7+
9
11
15+
16
17
18+
24
24+
25+
26
28
31+
32+
35+

the average value of the uncensored survival times reported as the mean survival time. This estimate is incorrect, since it ignores the information about the patients who remain alive. A mean of all times (both censored and not) is an underestimate, since the censored observations are really minimum possible survival times. However, it too, is often interpreted as the average survival time.

An alternative measure that may be meaningful is the survival probability at some time point of interest (e.g., at 2 years). How might this be computed? Using the data in Table 2.5, one measure would be $11/20 = 0.55$, based on the fact that 11 of 20 patients either died after 24 months (7), or were censored before 24 months (4). This probability is optimistic, since it assumes that all patients with censored observations less than 2 years would have survived a full 2 years if they had been observed further. Another approach would be to ignore those patients who were censored prior to 2 years, yielding a rate of $7/16 = 0.44$. This proportion was computed by deleting all patients who had censored observations prior to 24 months. This estimate is overly pessimistic, since it disregards information we do have about additional patient survival. A third approach that has been used in the literature is to ignore all patients (both alive and dead) who would not have been followed for at least 2 years. This, too, ignores valuable information.

Ideally, we wish to use as much patient information as possible. The most common method used in clinical trials is to estimate the survival experience of the patients using the Kaplan-Meier (product-limit) estimate (Kaplan and

TABLE 2.6

Calculation of Cumulative Survival Proportions for the Imaginary Trial Data

Time (Months)	# at Risk	# of Deaths	# Censored	Surviving This Time	Cumulative Survival
1	20	1	0	19/20 = 0.95	0.95
2	19	1	0	18/19	0.95 × (18/19) = 0.90
4	18	0	1	18/18	0.90 × (18/18) = 0.90
6	17	2	0	15/17	0.90 × (15/17) = 0.79
7	15	0	1	15/15	0.79 × (15/15) = 0.79
9	14	1	0	13/14	0.79 × (13/14) = 0.74
11	13	1	0	12/13	0.68[1]
15	12	0	1	12/12	0.68
16	11	1	0	10/11	0.62
17	10	1	0	9/10	0.56
18	9	0	1	9/9	0.56
24	8	1	1	7/8*	0.49
25	6	0	1	6/6	0.49
26	5	1	0	4/5	0.39
28	4	1	0	3/4	0.29
31	3	0	1	3/3	0.29
32	2	0	1	2/2	0.29
35	1	0	1	1/1	0.29

[1]The remaining cumulative survival estimates are calculated in the same way as the above calculations.

*Time at which both a death and a censored observation occured simultaneously.

Meier, 1958). The data from Table 2.5 are expanded in Table 2.6, with the addition of calculations of the survival curve. The second column of the table gives the number of patients alive just before the given time. This number represents the number of patients at risk of dying at the next observation time. The next two columns summarize how many patients die, or are censored. For each listed time the percent surviving is simply the ratio of the number remaining alive compared to the number at risk.

The final column lists the cumulative chance of surviving. At time zero, all patients are alive, and thus the initial cumulative percent of patients alive begins at 100%. At time 1, there is one death, and thus the proportion surviving, and the cumulative proportion surviving is 19/20, or 0.95. At the next time interval, there are now 19 patients still at risk (since one has already died). There is one death, giving a proportion surviving of 18/19 = 0.947. Cumulatively, the probability of surviving for 2 months is the product of the probability of surviving 1 month, times the probability of surviving 2 months among those surviving 1 month. Thus, this probability is estimated as 0.95 × 0.947 = 0.90 (which is just 18/20, the fraction surviving 2 months). At time 4, there are 18 patients at risk. One patient is censored at this point. Thus, the probability of surviving 4 months is 18/18 = 1, and the cumulative probability remains unchanged. However, in the next time interval, the patient with the censored observation at time 4 is no longer under observation, and is dropped from the number of patients at risk. Two patients die

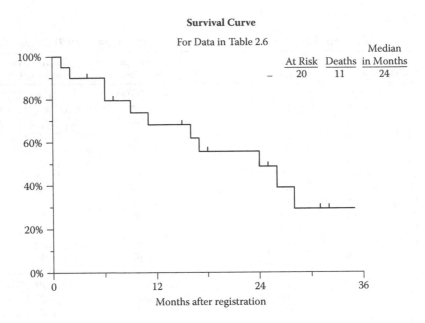

FIGURE 2.7
Plot of the survival curve calculated in Table 2.6.

at time 6, so that the estimate of the probability of surviving time 6 given survival past time 4 is $15/17 = 0.882$, and the cumulative chance of surviving 6 months is estimated by $0.90 \times 0.88 = 0.794$. Note that this is in between the value achieved by throwing the censored observation out of all calculations ($15/19 = 0.789$) and assuming that individual is still at risk past time 6 ($16/20 = 0.80$).

The estimated cumulative proportions surviving are calculated similarly for all observation times. The (*) in Table 2.6 indicates a time at which both a death and a censored observation occurred simultaneously. In calculating the estimate, we assume that the censored observation occurs after the death (in this case, just past 24 months), and hence is treated as being in a later time period. The successive products of the individual proportions surviving gives this estimate the name product-limit estimator. Using this technique, we obtain a 24-month survival estimate of 0.49.

A plot of the survival curve computed above is given in Figure 2.7. The curve is graphed as a step function, meaning it remains constant except at the death times. Statistically this is the most appropriate; attempting to interpolate between points can lead to biased estimates. The tic marks on the graph represent the censored observations.

We can now use this curve to provide point estimates of survival statistics of interest. For example, if 1-year survival is commonly reported, one would read up from the 12-month point on the horizontal axis, and find the estimated 1-year survival to be 0.68.

Instead of survival at some selected time, a common statistic of interest is the median survival time. This is the time at which one estimates that half of the patients will have died. The median survival time is estimated from the product-limit estimate to be the first time that the survival curve falls to 0.50 or below. For our example, the survival estimate is 0.56 at 17 months, and falls to 0.49 at 24 months. Thus the median survival is estimated to be 24 months.

Approximate confidence interval formulas are available for the product-limit estimates of the proportion surviving (Breslow and Crowley, 1972) and for the median survival (Brookmeyer and Crowley, 1982). What is most important to remember is that the width of the confidence intervals increases as one estimates further out on the time scale. This is because fewer patients contribute information as time increases. Thus, one will have more confidence in the accuracy of survival estimates from early in the Kaplan-Meier curve than for estimates from late in the curve. For example, if only two patients were entered on study longer than 5 years ago, the estimated 5-year survival probability is of questionable accuracy.

There are several common pitfalls in the interpretation of data from a survival curve. One common mistake is the attempt to interpret a final nonzero estimate of survival as a plateau. By the nature of the estimation procedure, if the final observation is a censored one, the survival curve will not reach zero. This does not imply that the probability of dying has ended, but rather that follow-up has run out. Related to this is the frequent extrapolation of the final cumulative survival past the times for which patients were observed. For example, in a study with data similar to those presented in Table 2.6, there is no information concerning the shape of the curve after 35 months.

Typically, in a Phase III clinical trial, we are not merely interested in estimating a survival curve. Our primary goal is to compare the survival curves between the treatment groups under study. Our hypotheses are usually formulated in terms of differences in survival, namely $H_o : S_A = S_B$ versus $S_B > S_A$, where S represents the true survival curve in the population. That is, our null hypothesis is that the two treatment regimens have the same survival, whereas the alternative is that the new treatment B improves survival over the standard treatment A. One approach taken has been to compare the survival curves at a single point, e.g., to compare the 2-year survival probabilities. Historically, this was done by estimating the probability in each group, and performing a test comparing these two probabilities. One problem with this is that the choice of the time point for testing is rather arbitrary. In addition, there are many situations for which the 2-year survival probabilities are the same, but the overall survival is very different. Figure 2.2b displays three situations, all giving rise to the same 2-year probabilities. One would usually prefer an overall test of the equality of the survival curves. There are a number of ways to do this. The general idea is the following: Begin by ordering the survival times (and censored observations), disregarding treatment assignment. Figure 2.8 gives several examples. In these, the A's represent deaths from patients receiving treatment arm A, and the B's are the deaths from

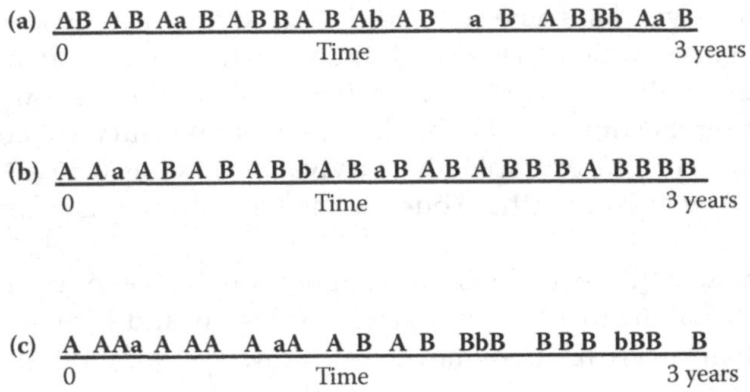

(a) <u>AB A B Aa B A B B A B Ab A B   a B   A B Bb Aa B</u>
    0   Time   3 years

(b) <u>A Aa AB A B AB bA B aB AB A BB B A BBBB</u>
    0   Time   3 years

(c) <u>A AAa A AA   A aA   A B A B   BbB   B B B bBB   B</u>
    0   Time   3 years

FIGURE 2.8
Patterns of survival times for two treatments (A and B represent true survival times, a and b represent censored observations).

patients receiving treatment arm B. The lower case values are the respective censored observations.

If there were no effect of treatment, we would expect that the deaths that came from arm A would occur over the whole range of death times, as would the deaths from arm B (Figure 2.8a). However, if there were a treatment difference, we would expect to see some pattern, such as those seen in Figures 2.8b and c.

We can set up a test as follows. Each observation is assigned a score such as an ordered rank, with the earliest death given rank 1, the second rank 2, etc. If there is no difference in survival, we would expect that the deaths from the patients in arm A would have some small and some large scores, as would the patients in arm B. However, if there are differences in the groups (one has more deaths, or all of the deaths are earlier), then we'd expect that one group would have more of the large (or small) scores. We can use the difference in the sum of the scores from the two groups as a test statistic. There are a number of common test statistics for censored data, each of which differ in the way the scores are determined. The most common is called the logrank test (Mantel, 1966); other test statistics are given by Gehan (1965), Peto and Peto (1972), and Prentice (1978). As for the χ^2 test for discrete data, p-values can be computed for the calculated value of the logrank test for the purpose of testing the null hypothesis of equal survival in the two treatment groups.

An alternative explanation of censored data test statistics starts with 2×2 tables similar to those in Section 2.3.1. Consider the data in Table 2.7, taken from Figure 2.8a. All the survival times have been ordered, ignoring treatment arm and whether or not the observations are censored.

At the time of each uncensored observation (death times), a 2×2 table is formed. The marginal totals are the number alive in each arm just before that time (the number at risk), the number who die at that time, and the number who survive, and the cell entries are the number dying and the number surviving in each arm. The notation is shown in Table 2.8.

TABLE 2.7

Survival Times (in Months) for Treatments A and B

Time (months)	Arm
1	A
2	B
4+	B
6	A
6	A
7+	A
9	B
11	B
15+	A
16	B
17	B
18+	A
24	A
24+	B
25+	A
26	B
28	B
31+	A
32+	B
35+	A

For example, at time 11 in Table 2.7, $n_A = 6$, $n_B = 7$, $d_A = 0$, and $d_B = 1$. The observed number of deaths in arm A is d_A, and the expected number under H_0, the null hypothesis of no difference, is $n_A d/n$. Define the quantity $V = n_A n_B d(n-d)/n^2(n-1)$, which is the denominator in one of the derivations of the χ^2 statistic in Section 2.3.1. For survival data measured in small units of time such as days, the number d dying at a time t will be 1, so that V reduces to $n_A n_B/n^2$. Then the logrank test is defined as $[\sum(d_A - n_A d/n)]^2 / \sum V$, where the sum is over all of the times of death. With this notation, other test statistics can be defined by weighting the summands in the numerator differently: $[\sum w(d_A - n_A d/n)]^2 / \sum V$.

For example, the Gehan (1965) version of the Wilcoxon test puts more weight on earlier deaths than on later ones ($w = n$, the total number at risk),

TABLE 2.8

2 × 2 Table at a Death Time t

	Deaths	Survivors	Total at Risk
Arm A	d_A	$n_A - d_A$	n_A
Arm B	d_B	$n_B - d_B$	n_B
Totals	d	$n - d$	n

while the logrank test weighs each table equally. The Peto and Peto (1972) and Prentice (1978) test statistics mentioned earlier also fit this formulation, with weight w being (roughly) the value of the product-limit estimate from the combined sample at time t (and thus giving more weight to earlier deaths). For more details, see for example Crowley and Breslow, 1984. The ambitious reader can check that the value of the logrank test statistic for the data in Table 2.7 is 0.60, which when referred to tables of the χ^2 distribution gives a p-value of 0.44. (Remember to order the censored time at 24 months as just larger than the uncensored time).

Although the most efficient Phase III trial is designed to compare only two treatments, some trials are designed with three or more treatment arms. There is a natural extension of the logrank test (and χ^2 test) that can accommodate this situation. If the null hypothesis is that there is no survival difference (or difference in response) among any of the K groups, and the alternative hypothesis is that some differences in survival (response) exist, then a single test is performed. If the null hypothesis of complete equality is rejected, then secondary analyses are performed to identify the source of the difference. Separate comparisons between all combinations of treatment pairs, without a preliminary test or other statistical adjustment, are inappropriate and should be avoided. Performing these "multiple comparisons" results in an overall Type I error (the probability of concluding there is a difference in **any** of these pairwise comparisons when there are no treatment differences) that is higher than the level of each individual test. There are several techniques for avoiding this problem of multiple comparisons (see Chapter 6).

2.4 The Proportional Hazards Model

So far we have concentrated on estimation of the proportion alive (or dead) at various times. Now we turn to a different characteristic of the survival distribution, introduced in Section 2.1, the hazard function. Although exponential distributions (with a constant hazard rate λ) are commonly used for such purposes as sample size calculation, most often we have no idea what form the underlying hazard function, more generally denoted $\lambda(t)$, will take. No matter what that form, in Phase III trials we are usually most interested in comparing the hazards between the treatment arms (this is equivalent to comparing the survival curves). As part of that comparison, we often wish to assess whether the difference, if any, that we observe, could be due to differences among the patients in important prognostic factors. For example, if there were more high-risk patients in one treatment arm than the other, we would like to know whether any survival differences were due to the high-risk patients as opposed to a true treatment effect. In order to answer these questions, a statistical model has been developed which is an extension of the logrank test designed to accommodate other variables of interest. This model is called the Cox regression model (Cox, 1972), or the proportional hazards model. This model assumes that the hazard function for each patient is the product of some general hazard function multiplied by a term related to patient characteristics and other prognostic factors of interest. Mathematically, this function is described by

$$\lambda(t, x_i) = (\lambda_0(t)) \exp\left(\sum_i \beta_i x_i\right),$$

or equivalently

$$\ln(\lambda(t, x_i)) = \ln(\lambda_0(t)) + \left(\sum_i \beta_i x_i\right),$$

where $\lambda(t, x_i)$ is the hazard function for the patient, x_i describes the covariates for that patient, and the β's are regression coefficients. For example, when the only covariate is treatment, coded say as $x = 0$ for treatment A and $x = 1$ for treatment B, this model states that the hazard functions for the two treatments are given by $\lambda_0(t)$ and $\lambda_0(t) \exp(\beta)$, respectively. The ratio of these hazard functions is for all t the constant $\exp(\beta)$; thus the name "proportional hazards model." The proportional hazards model can be used much as linear regression is used in other contexts, to assess the importance of prognostic factors and to compare treatments adjusted for such factors (see Chapters 8 and 10). It can account for both categorical variables, such as treatment arm assignment and sex, and for continuous measurements such as age and CA-125. The logrank test can be derived from the model when there are no covariates other than treatment; a generalization of the logrank test, adjusted for covariates, results from the larger model.

It is important to note that the proportional hazards model imposes no requirements on the form of the hazard functions, only on their ratios. An important generalization that makes even fewer assumptions is the stratified Cox model. For example, it may be that the hazard functions for covariates can not be assumed to be proportional, but adjustment for covariates still needs to be made in a test for differences between two treatments. In this case one can define proportional hazards models for treatment, within strata defined by levels of the covariates (continuous covariates can be reduced to categories for this purpose). The model is

$$\lambda_j(t, x) = (\lambda_{0j}(t)) \exp(\beta x),$$

where j indexes the strata and x identifies the treatment group. Use of this model does not allow for the assessment of whether the stratifying covariates are important with regard to survival, but it does allow for adjusted treatment comparisons, and in fact leads to what is termed the stratified logrank test.

2.5 Sample Size Calculations

Earlier in the chapter we alluded to the relationship among level, power, magnitude of differences to detect, and sample size. In this section, we discuss the issues involved in estimation of sample size for clinical trials, and present one technique used in sample size determination.

Recall that there are three quantities related to sample size: level, power, and a difference one wishes to detect. Computer programs and tables exist for determining sample size estimates. It is useful, however, to consider a sample size formula, in order to understand how the above quantities interrelate. The derivation for these formulas can be found in standard statistical texts (see, for example, Fleiss, 1981) and will not be presented here.

When the outcomes are dichotomous, such as response collapsed into CR + PR versus others, the following formula can be used to obtain sample size estimates for the comparison of two treatment arms. Let p_A be the hypothesized response probability in arm A, and p_B be the response probability one hopes to detect in arm B. The average of these two probabilities is given by $\bar{p} = (p_A + p_B)/2$. The formula is

$$N = \frac{\left(z_\alpha\sqrt{2\bar{p}(1-\bar{p})} + z_\beta\sqrt{p_A(1-p_A) + p_B(1-p_B)}\right)^2}{(p_A - p_B)^2}, \qquad (2.1)$$

where N is the required sample size for each treatment arm, z_α is the value for which $F(z_\alpha) = 1 - \alpha$, and z_β is the value for which $F(z_\beta) = 1 - \beta$, and $F(z)$ is the normal distribution. For $\alpha = 0.05$, $z_\alpha = 1.645$ for a one-sided test, and $z_\alpha = 1.96$ for a two-sided test. If a power of 90% is desired, then $\beta = (1 - 0.9) = 0.1$, and $z_\beta = 1.282$.

From the above formula, note that the quantity in the denominator is the difference in the response probabilities for the two treatments. The smaller this denominator is, the larger the resulting N will be. Thus, if one wishes to be able to detect a relatively small treatment effect, a larger sample size will be required than if one is only interested in detecting large differences in the treatments. Similarly, if one wishes to have greater power (causing z_β to be larger) or smaller significance level (causing z_α to be larger), the numerator will be larger, also increasing the required sample size. The numerator and thus the sample size are also larger when p_A and p_B are closer to 0.5 than to 0 or 1, since the maximum value of $p(1 - p)$ is 0.25 when $p = 0.5$, and the minimum is 0 when p is 0 or 1. Table 2.9 presents the total sample size $2N$ required to detect selected choices of response probabilities in a two-arm clinical trial. (A slightly different formula from 2.1, due to Fleiss et al., 1980, was used.)

The table illustrates the fact that for a fixed difference $\Delta = p_B - p_A$, the sample size increases as p_A moves from 0.1 toward 0.5. For example, if $p_A = 0.1$, the total sample size is 80 to detect an increase of 0.3; however, if $p_A = 0.3$, the required total sample size is 104.

TABLE 2.9

Total Sample Size $2N$ Required to Detect an Increase in p_A by Δ for Significance Level 0.05, Power 0.90, One-Sided Test

p_A	$\Delta = 0.1$	$\Delta = 0.15$	$\Delta = 0.2$	$\Delta = 0.25$	$\Delta = 0.3$
0.1	472	242	152	108	80
0.2	678	326	196	132	96
0.3	816	380	222	146	104
0.4	884	402	230	148	104

When the outcome is survival, we usually make the simplifying assumption that survival follows an exponential distribution. Formulas similar in spirit to 2.1 above, though more complicated, are used to estimate the required sample size for trials of this type. A discussion of sample size for a two-arm trial with survival as the endpoint is contained in Section 6.1.

2.6 Concluding Remarks

There is an important distinction between a clinically significant difference and a statistically significant difference. Any numerical difference, no matter how small (and possibly of minimal, if any clinical interest) can yield a statistically significant test if the sample size is sufficiently large.

This chapter has introduced key statistical concepts and analyses. Understanding the basics will help in understanding why statisticians choose specific designs and analyses in specific settings. These choices are the subject of the rest of the book.

3

The Design of Clinical Trials

Then Daniel said to the steward whom the chief of the eunuchs had appointed over Daniel, "Test your servants for ten days; let us be given vegetables to eat and water to drink. Then let our appearance and the appearance of the youths who eat the king's rich food be observed by you, and according to what you see deal with your servants." So he hearkened to them in this matter, and tested them for ten days. At the end of ten days it was seen that they were better in appearance and fatter in flesh than all the youths who ate the king's rich food. So the steward took away their rich food and the wine they were to drink, and gave them vegetables.

—**Daniel 1: 11-16**

It has been suggested that the biblical dietary comparison introducing the chapter is the first clinical trial in recorded history, and its designer, Daniel, the first trialist (Fisher, 1983). In this chapter, we introduce important elements of designing a clinical trial. Specifics for design of Phase I, II, and III trials are discussed in Chapters 4, 5, and 6, respectively.

The major elements in designing a clinical trial are

1. Stating the objectives clearly,
2. Specifying eligibility,
3. Specifying treatment arms, including choice of an appropriate control,
4. Specifying how treatment assignment will be accomplished for randomized comparative trials, including a decision as to whether blinding is necessary,
5. Specifying endpoints, including a decision as to whether independent review is required,
6. Determining the magnitude of difference to be detected or the desired precision of estimation, and identifying other assumptions to be used for the design,
7. Deciding whether an independent data monitoring committee is required, and if so, the composition, and
8. Ethical considerations.

3.1 Objectives

Identifying the primary objective requires careful thought about what key conclusions are to be made at the end of the trial. The statement "To compare A and B," for instance, is not a sufficient statement of objectives. Is the goal to identify one of the arms for further study? To reach a definitive conclusion about which arm to use in the future to treat a specific type of patient? To decide if addition of a new agent improves treatment outcome? To determine if A and B are equivalent? To generate evidence for or against a biologic hypothesis? Each of these objectives has different design implications. For the first, a relatively small randomized Phase II selection design might be appropriate. The second and third require a reasonably large randomized trial, with two-sided superiority testing for the first and one-sided for the second. The fourth needs a larger sample size and a focus on precise estimation. The fifth might require interaction testing and require an even larger sample size. (See Chapters 5 and 6 for design specifics.)

3.2 Eligibility

The eligibility criteria must be suitable for the stated objectives. Consideration should be given to which patients are likely to benefit from treatment and to the desired generalizability of results. If eligibility criteria are very narrow, the generalizability of the study is compromised; if they are too broad, the effectiveness of treatment may be masked by inclusion of patients with little chance of benefiting. For instance, some Phase II studies are not reproducible because they were restricted to very good risk patients. On the other hand, other Phase II studies can be unduly negative because they were conducted in heavily pretreated patients who would not be expected to respond to therapy.

Including very disparate groups of patients (e.g., more than one type of cancer or more than one line of treatment) and hoping to sort out which types benefit at the end of the trial is usually not a good strategy. Trials generally are designed to detect a benefit over all in the population accrued and have limited power for testing subset results. (See Chapter 9 for a discussion of the pitfalls of subset analyses.) On the other hand, some newer designs are specifically aimed at exploring different histological types, where there may be similarities across subtypes which can be exploited (LeBlanc et al., 2009).

The recent emphasis on targeted agents brings new challenges to this issue. It is anticipated that a subset of patients with specific disease characteristics will benefit most from treatment, but it may not be well understood which characteristics are most predictive of benefit. Stewart et al. (2010) point out that large trials are conducted to overcome the fact that only a small subset of patients benefit from treatment, which results either in loss of benefit to the subset (if the trial fails) or over-treatment of most patients (if the trial does not). Thus trial designs may need to explicitly accommodate exploratory biology aims as well as treatment comparisons. (See Chapters 4–6 and 10 for discussion on how these might be addressed.)

3.3 Treatment Arms

Usefulness of an experimental treatment typically is assessed against either a specific control arm or against expected results from the literature. For the assessment to be valid, the comparator treatment must be as similar as possible with the exception of the aspect of treatment being tested. For instance, if the primary aim of a trial of agent C alone versus a combination of agents C and D is to decide whether the addition of agent D improves the effectiveness of agent C, then the administration of agent C should be identical on the two treatment arms; otherwise differences could be due to alterations in C as well as to the addition of D. If a dose question is being addressed, the number of cycles and cycle length on each arm should be the same; otherwise differences could be due to duration or intensity of treatment instead of dose. If the aim is to demonstrate that regimen A should become the new standard of care, then regimen B should be the current standard of care, not a variation on standard or another experimental regimen; otherwise B may be suspected as potentially worse than standard.

3.3.1 Single Arm

For single-arm trials all patients receive the same treatment and results are assessed against expected results based on previous historical experience. The patient population from which the historic estimate is based should have similar patient characteristics, similar standard of care and use the same diagnostic and screening procedures as patients anticipated to be entered onto the new study. In addition, the primary outcome should be objective and consistently defined so that results from the trial have the same interpretation as for results from the historical control. Unfortunately, an estimate for the population to be used in a current study may not be available, and even if one is, historical estimates for apparently the same treatment and same patient population may vary substantially. Studies allow for a range of patients to be entered and the mix may not be comparable despite the same eligibility criteria. This makes it difficult to choose an appropriate value against which the new treatment should be assessed.

Consider the following example illustrating how reference to a historical control can be misleading. Pérol et al., reported on a Phase II trial of alternating chemotherapy in first line therapy for advanced non-small-cell lung cancer. The primary endpoint was objective response, with a primary aim to decide whether to test in a Phase III trial versus control. A typical single-arm assessment of alternating therapy using a two-stage design with the null hypothesis $H_0 = 0.30$ was planned. A randomized control group was included to "calibrate" the study population and a reference response of 0.43 based on a recent Phase III study was stated. The estimated response probability for the alternating regimen was a dismal 0.11. However, the estimate on the control arm was only 0.25, significantly lower than the referenced 0.43, so it is clear that the trial null hypothesis was inappropriate for the population accrued. For this study it was still reasonable to conclude the experimental regimen should not be studied further (in addition to having a low response estimate it was toxic), but the example does illustrate that active regimens might be missed if the historical control information does not apply.

Single-arm trials are most appropriate if historical estimates are well characterized, consistent, and have been stable over time. For cancers with uniformly low probability of success this approach may be feasible. However, recent advances have reduced the settings in which the classical single-arm Phase IIs are easily applied. Other trial designs are becoming more common, particularly as new subtypes of disease are being identified and addressed, and as previously poor success rates improve. (See Chapter 5 for Phase II design options.)

3.3.2 Two or More Treatment Arms

Comparative trials with control groups consisting of a specific set of past patients are sometimes designed. Alternatively patients may be entered onto a trial nonrandomly, e.g., all A followed by all B or alternating A and B. A carefully chosen specific group of previous patients or sets of patients managed on the same trial could potentially be better choices for comparison than an estimate from the literature, but will still be subject to biases since many of the factors that lead to the selection of treatments by patients and physicians will be unavailable or unknown. (See Chapter 9 for examples of the pitfalls of historical controls.)

In cases of a limited patient population a trial using a previous set of patients for the comparison may be the only feasible option. As for single-arm trials, care must be taken to choose a comparator with characteristics as similar as possible to the new patients to be studied. See Chapter 5 for further discussion of two arm nonrandomized trials.

Randomized trials may consist of one or more standard treatments, or a control treatment arm and one or more experimental treatment arms. Depending on standard of care, the control arm may consist of no treatment, a placebo, or standard active therapy with or without a placebo (Food and Drug Administration, 2001). Details of randomized Phase II trials are discussed in Chapter 5, and Phase III trials in Chapter 6.

3.4 Randomized Treatment Assignment

Randomization ensures that patients are assigned to treatment arms without systematic differences in baseline characteristics. It is the cornerstone of clinical trials methodology. Without it, we would still be in the dark ages of observational studies, with no satisfactory way to assess whether any improvements observed were due to the treatment being studied or to selection factors. It now seems foolish that it was thought that patients got better because of—rather than in spite of—purging, bleeding, and blistering, but recent history has hardly been free of observational misinterpretations. Was the unquestioned use of radical mastectomy for so many years much different? Or, until randomized studies were done, was it just another untested procedure predicated on an incorrect theory of a disease process?

Randomization isn't quite sufficient by itself to guarantee that treatment arms will be balanced with respect to patient characteristics, unless the sample size is large. In small- or moderate-size studies imbalances in important patient characteristics can occur by chance and compromise interpretation of the study (Redman and Crowley, 2007). It is prudent to protect against this possibility by making sure the most important factors are reasonably well balanced between the arms. Patient characteristics incorporated into the randomization scheme to achieve balance are called stratification factors. See Chapter 6 for a discussion of randomization schemes.

Randomization doesn't work if patients are routinely "canceled" after entry on trial. If investigators and patients proceed with treatment assignments only if the randomization is to a preferred arm, then the trial is little better than a study on patients who were treated according to systematic non-random reasons. Due to the selection biases introduced by cancellation, all randomized trials should be conducted according to the intent-to-treat principle (see Chapter 8).

3.4.1 Blinding

Randomization is necessary for controlling selection bias but does not guarantee the final comparison will be unbiased. There are numerous potential sources of bias that can occur after randomization and to the extent these biases differ according to treatment group, the treatment comparison is compromised. For instance, when patients know they are on a control arm they may not be motivated to return for outcome assessments or may discontinue the study to receive non-protocol treatment. Investigators may be less likely to attribute adverse events to control treatment than to experimental or may take control patients off treatment at earlier signs of failure.

Blinded placebo controlled trials are done to reduce the potential for biases related to knowledge of treatment assignment. For patients, compliance is enhanced and supplemental treatments, while not necessarily eliminated, should at least be balanced across the groups. For investigators, objectivity of outcome assessments is improved. "Double-blinding" means that neither the patient nor the clinician knows what treatment has been assigned to the patient. "Single-blinding" means only the patient doesn't know. "Placebo-controlled" means patients on all arms receive identical-appearing treatment, but all or part of the treatment is inactive on one of the arms. Blinded, placebo-controlled trials are the most rigorous and convincing type of randomized trial, but they are expensive. Manufacture of placebos, labeling of active and inactive treatment with code numbers and keeping track of them, shipping supplies of coded treatments, communications with the pharmacies that dispense the treatments, mechanisms for unblinding in medical emergencies all are time consuming to plan and costly to administer. There are various circumstances when blinded trials are necessary, but consider the difficulties carefully before embarking on one. One necessary circumstance is when treatment on one of the arms is commercially available (e.g., vitamins). In this case it is important for compliance that patients on each arm get an identical-appearing pill and that all patients are blinded to their assignments. This should minimize and equalize the number of patients who obtain their own supply of active drug. Whether or not the clinicians also need to be blinded depends on whether knowledge of assignment will lead to inappropriate alterations of treatment or to biased assessments.

Placebos and double-blinding are also necessary when important endpoints are subjective, due to the well-known placebo effect (Shapiro and Shapiro, 1997). Patients frequently feel better or experience side effects in anticipation of receiving active treatment. For instance, in a double-blind antiemetic trial of placebo versus prochlorperazine (PCP) versus tetrahydrocannabinol (THC) (Frytak et al., 1979), the percent of patients on the treatment arms reported as having sedation as a side effect were high—71% on prochlorperazine and 76% on THC. Without a placebo comparison, the 71% and 76% might have been judged against 0% and the side effect judged excessive. As it was, sedation was reported in 46% of placebo patients. Coordination problems were reported for 19% of placebo patients (3% "intolerable"), and "highs" were reported in 12% of PCP patients. THC had significantly higher percentages of these two effects, but without a double blind comparison, the results could have been criticized as reflecting biased assessments rather than true differences. Both THC and PCP had significant antiemetic effects compared to placebo. Overall unsatisfactory outcome (either repeated vomiting or CNS side effects requiring discontinuation of treatment) was reported as 54%, 46%, and 63%, respectively, for placebo, PCP, and THC (nonsignificant). Interestingly, the paper concludes THC should not be recommended for general use, but makes no comment on the usefulness of PCP.

Blinding can't always be achieved even if considered necessary. For instance, blinding doesn't work if the active treatment has a distinctive side effect. Occurrence of the side effect will effectively unblind the treatment arm and biased assessments of all endpoints may result. The limited information available on effectiveness of blinding suggests mixed success. Hróbjartsson et al. (2007) did a review of publications of blinded studies. Only 31 reported on how well the blinding worked and of these only 14 were reported as successful. Assessment of blinding is tricky. One might assume that if more than 50% of patients on a two arm trial guess correctly then blinding failed. This is not necessarily correct. For instance, if everyone who has a response guesses they were on the experimental arm regardless and everyone without a response guesses they were on control, then if the experimental arm is effective more than 50% of guesses will be correct independent of whether the blind was broken (Boutron et al., 2005).

If a blinded trial is done, decisions must be made as to the timing and conditions for unblinding. Unblinding is clearly necessary in medical emergencies in which treatment depends on knowledge of trial assignment. Otherwise it is best not to unblind anyone until the study is complete. Risks of early knowledge of treatment assignment include patients who had been on placebo deciding to take active treatment, and clinicians receiving enough clues to be able to recognize treatment assignment in patients supposedly still on blinded treatment, leading to biased assessments of subjective endpoints.

3.5 Endpoints

Endpoints must be suitable for the objectives. For instance, if the primary aim is to identify the arm of choice for treating patients, then endpoints that best reflect benefit to the patient should be used. Tumor shrinkage in itself usually is not of direct benefit to a patient, whereas longer survival or symptom improvement is. Using convenient or short-term endpoints instead of the ones of primary interest can result in incorrect conclusions. (See Chapter 9 for a discussion of surrogate endpoints.)

Many of the common endpoints used in clinical trials are problematic in one way or another, often due to correlation among possible outcomes or due to the logical traps in complicated definitions. The examples below are commonly used endpoints in cancer trials, but the same principles hold for endpoints for any clinical study.

3.5.1 Survival

Survival is defined as the time from registration on study to time of death due to any cause. As described in Chapter 2, survival distributions can still be estimated when not all patients have died by using the information from "censored" survival times (time from registration to date of last contact for living patients) as well as from the known death times.

Survival is the most straightforward and objective of cancer endpoints, but even here there can be problems. Bias can result when there are many patients lost to follow-up; examples are given in Section 3.7.1. If most patients are still alive at the time of analysis, estimates can be highly variable or not even defined. If many patients die of causes other than the cancer under study the interpretation of survival can be problematic, since the effect of treatment on the disease under study is of primary interest.

Using time to death due to disease (defined the same way as survival, except that observations are censored at the time of death if death is due to causes other than the cancer of interest) is not a solution to the problem of competing causes of death. Even if cause of death information is reliable, which is often not the case, unbiased estimation of time to death due to disease is possible only if deaths due to other causes are statistically independent of the cancer being studied, and if it makes sense to think of "removing" the risk of dying from other causes. (See Chapter 9 for a discussion of competing risks.) The independence of causes of death is rarely a good assumption. Good and poor risk cancer patients tend to be systematically different with respect to susceptibility to other potentially lethal diseases as well as to their cancers. Furthermore, the cause specific endpoint does not include all effects of treatment on survival. Examples of other effects include early toxic deaths, late deaths due to leukemia after treatment with alkylating agents, death due to congestive heart failure after treatment with Adriamycin, etc. These examples all represent failures of treatment. Since it is not possible to tell which causes of death are or are not related to the disease or its treatment, or what the nature of the relationships might be, it is not possible to tell exactly what "time to death due to disease" estimates. Furthermore, if results using this endpoint are different from those using overall survival, the latter must take precedence. (A treatment generally isn't going to be considered effective if deaths due to disease are decreased only at the expense of increased deaths due to other causes.) We recommend using only overall survival.

3.5.2 Progression-Free Survival (PFS)

Progression-free survival (or relapse-free survival for adjuvant studies) is defined as the time from registration to the first observation of disease progression or death due to any cause. If a patient has not progressed or died, progression-free survival is censored at the time of last follow-up or at the time of last disease assessment (if the last follow-up occurs long after the last disease assessment, bias may be introduced). This endpoint is preferred to time to progression (with censorship at the time of death if the death is due to other causes) for reasons similar to those noted above. A problem with PFS is that the time of progression is not known exactly but rather known only to lie in the interval between disease assessments (leading to interval censored observations). This means that estimates of PFS depend on the assessment schedule, and that standardization of assessment schedules across randomized arms is necessary for unbiased comparisons. Another problem we find with the progression-free survival endpoint is that advanced disease is often not followed for progression after a patient has been taken off treatment for toxicity or refusal. Since early discontinuation of treatment in advanced disease typically is related to poor patient response or tolerance, in these studies we sometimes use failure-free survival (time from registration to the first observation of disease progression, death due to any cause, or early discontinuation of treatment). If, instead, results are censored at time of discontinuation then there is a good chance of introducing bias. Typically one would expect the resulting estimates to be optimistic, but this cannot be assumed. For instance, some patients may discontinue if they are feeling well and want a break from treatment. This kind of informative censoring is even more of an issue when PFS is judged centrally (and retrospectively). When a local progression is not verified centrally, subsequent scans are rarely available for additional review, leading to a number of patients being censored at the time the treating investigator judged the patient to be failing. This would be anticipated to result in an optimistic bias in the PFS estimate. Dodd et al., 2008, examine the utility of independent central review and conclude that double blinding is the best approach to minimize bias. Since central review can introduce bias instead of reducing it, PFS by central review is not recommended as the primary endpoint when double blinding is possible.

A variation on progression-free survival is duration of response, defined as the time from first observation of response to the first time of progression or death. If a responding patient has not progressed, duration of response is censored at the time of last follow-up or at the time of last disease assessment. Since it can be misleading to report failure times only in a subset of patients, particularly when the subset is chosen based on another outcome, we don't recommend use of this endpoint. (Chapter 9 gives more details on this issue.)

3.5.3 Response

Response in the past was typically defined as a 50% decrease in bidimensionally measurable disease lasting 4 weeks, progression as a 25% increase in any lesion, relapse as a 50% increase in responding disease. We were often assured that everyone knew what this meant, but found that what everyone knew varied quite a lot. For instance, does a patient with a 25% increase in one lesion at the same time as a 50% decrease in the sum of products of perpendicular diameters of all measurable lesions have a response or not? Is the 25% increase measured from baseline, or from the minimum size? If it is an increase over baseline, does it make sense that a lesion which shrinks to $1.4 \text{ cm} \times 1.5 \text{ cm}$ from 2×2 must increase to 2.24×2.24 to be a progression, while one which shrinks to 1.4×1.4 must only increase to 1.72×1.72 to be a relapse? In practice, is an increase in a previously unchanged lesion from 0.8×0.8 to 0.9×0.9 really treated as evidence of progression? If disease is documented to have decreased by 50% once, can it be assumed the decrease lasted 4 weeks, or does it have to be documented again? If nonmeasurable disease is clearly increasing, while measurable disease is decreasing, is this still a response? The previous standard SWOG response definition (Green and Weiss, 1992) was quite detailed in order to clarify these and other common ambiguities in response definitions.

Recognition of these and other issues led to an international collaboration to revise the World Health Organization response criteria. Over several years members of the European Organization for Research and Treatment of Cancer (EORTC), the National Cancer Institute of the United States and the National Cancer Institute of Canada Clinical Trials Group developed and published (Therasse et al., 2000) new criteria called RECIST (Response Evaluation Criteria in Solid Tumors). Many previously unaddressed aspects of response assessment were clarified. Additionally, a key modification implemented in these definitions was the change to unidimensional measurements instead of bidimensional. Assessments of various data sets indicated the simpler definition of 30% decrease in sum of maximum diameters resulted in very similar response determinations as the old 50% decrease in sum of products. (Note: If an M × M lesion decreases to 0.7 M × 0.7 M, then there is a 30% decrease in the maximum diameter and a 51% decrease in the product of diameters.) The change to 20% increase for progression resulted in somewhat longer time to progression in 7% of patients and shorter in 1%, but the differences were considered acceptable. (Note: If an M × M lesion increases to 1.2 M × 1.2 M, this is a 20% increase in maximum diameter and a 44% increase in product of diameters.) A recent update to RECIST was published addressing some remaining issues (Eisenhauer et al., 2009). The most significant change is to assessment of lymph nodes. Instead of the maximum diameter for a target node, the short diameter is measured and added to the sum of maximum diameters of other target lesions. If the node measurement decreases to < 10mm the node is considered normal and disease may be assessed as a CR if all other disease has disappeared. Note also a welcome suggestion from RECIST 1.1 that confirmation of response after 4 weeks is not necessary for randomized trials when response is not the primary endpoint, resulting in some simplification of trial conduct.

Despite standardizations, response remains a problematic endpoint. Nonmeasurable disease is hard to incorporate objectively, as is symptomatic deterioration without objective evidence of progression. Both problems introduce subjective judgment into response assessment. Furthermore, tests and scans are not all done on the same schedule (some infrequently), and due to cost constraints noncritical assessments may be skipped. This results in insufficient information to apply the strict definitions of response, either leaving final response determination as indeterminate or introducing even more subjective judgment. While response frequently is used as an indicator of biologic activity in Phase II studies (for which response monitoring tends to be more carefully done), it is not recommended as the primary endpoint in Phase III trials.

3.5.4 Toxicity Criteria

Toxicity endpoints also present a variety of logical problems. Toxicities are usually graded on a 6-point scale, from grade 0 (none) to grade 5 (fatal), with mild, moderate, severe, and life-threatening in between. Toxicities that cannot be life-threatening shouldn't have the highest grades defined. For instance, complete alopecia used to be categorized as grade 4; this is now more suitably included in grade 2. Lesser grades also should not be defined if they are not appropriate (cerebral necrosis would not be mild, for example). Care must be taken with the boundary values when categorizing continuous values into this discrete scale, so that there is no ambiguity (If grade 1 is $< x$ and grade 2 is $> x$, how is x categorized?). All the possibilities must be covered (If grade 1 is "mild and brief pain" and grade 2 is "severe and prolonged pain," how is a severe but brief pain classified?) and each possibility should be covered only once (If grade 1 is "mild or brief pain" and grade 2 is "severe or prolonged pain," severe but brief pain still can not be coded.). SWOG developed detailed toxicity criteria (Green and Weiss, 1992) to address such issues and to supplement the limited list of Common Toxicity Criteria (CTC) provided by the NCI. Since then, extensive changes and additions to the CTC (now termed Common Terminology Criteria for Adverse Events—CTCAE) have been developed and are in widespread use. The latest version can be found on the website of the Cancer Therapy Evaluation Program of NCI, currently http://ctep.cancer.gov/reporting/ctc.html.

3.5.5 Quality of Life

Quality of life is the hardest of cancer endpoints to assess. In the past, toxicity and response have often been used as surrogates for quality of life. Toxicity certainly reflects one aspect of quality (with the exception of abnormal lab values without symptoms), but response, by itself, may not. A response is not necessarily accompanied by benefits such as symptom relief or improvement in function; nor is an objective tumor response necessary for such benefits. There are many facets of quality of life, and the relative importance of each is a matter of individual preference. Physical and emotional functioning, plus general and treatment-specific symptoms have been identified as key aspects of quality of life in cancer patients. Another key to quality of life assessment is patient self-report. It's nice if physicians believe their patients are feeling better; it's even better if the patients think so. Detailed recommendations concerning quality of life assessment that have been implemented in SWOG have been published (Moinpour et al., 1989). However, proper assessment of quality of life is very expensive so it is not routinely incorporated into our studies (see Chapter 7). In addition, analysis of quality of life endpoints is challenging due to substantial amounts of missing data (see Chapter 8).

The message to take away from Section 3.5 is that endpoint definitions require careful attention. Imprecisely defined or subjective endpoints result in inconsistent or biased interpretation by investigators, which in turn result in a compromised interpretation of the study. On the other hand, precisely defined but inappropriate endpoints result in comparisons that don't answer the questions posed by the study. Choose wisely.

3.6 Differences to be Detected or Precision of Estimates and Other Assumptions

Although historical information cannot be used for definitive treatment comparisons, it is useful in specifying the assumptions required for sample size calculations. Estimates of characteristics of the endpoints (most often summary statistics such as the median, mean, standard deviation etc.) are needed, as is an estimate of the rate of accrual of patients. Other assumptions are also made, such as the typical proportional hazards assumption used to describe the difference in survival or progression-free survival between arms (see Chapter 2). It may be worth considering whether there is evidence that this standard assumption is suitable for the particular disease under study, as power may be reduced if the assumption is incorrect. For adjuvant breast cancer studies, for instance, disease-free survival hazard ratios may not be proportional, but rather decrease over time.

If a Phase III trial is planned, the trial generally should be designed to have sufficient power to detect the smallest difference that is clinically meaningful. A study is doomed to failure if it is designed to have good power to detect only unrealistically large differences. In practice, trials are often designed to have adequate power only to detect the smallest affordable difference, not the smallest meaningful difference. Consideration should be given as to whether the affordable difference is plausible enough to warrant doing the study at all, since it is a waste of resources to do a trial with little chance of yielding a definitive conclusion. Specifics for Phase III trial designs are discussed in Chapter 6.

A frequent point of confusion in designing trials concerns the difference between the alternative for which the study has power versus the difference that must be observed for a significant result. If the study is designed to test a null hypothesis of difference $= 0$ with adequate power for an alternative of difference $= x$, then the observed value needed to reject is not x. It will be around $x/2$. If you insist on seeing x instead of $x/2$ for a convincing result, then when x is true your power will be 50%—because when x is true then half the time the result is expected to be over x and half the time under. If you want a high chance of concluding the study is positive when x is true then values below x that are consistent with x being true will have to be included. Remember also that the conclusion when a result is positive is that the difference is greater than 0, not that the difference is x. We do not recommend that trials be designed with the observed result in mind, but if there is a concern that the observed difference at the end of a trial will not be viewed as clinically useful, then the only option is increase x (or equivalently, reduce power).

If a Phase II study is being designed, consideration should be given to how precise the results must be for the information to be useful. If the confidence interval for an estimate is so large that it covers the range of values from wonder drug to dud, then the information to be gained is not particularly useful, and the conduct of the trial should be discouraged. Specifics for Phase II trial designs are included in Chapter 5.

3.7 Use of Independent Data Monitoring Committees

If investigators are shown early results of trials, they might decide not to participate anymore for a variety of reasons. If trends are emerging, the current best arm might be considered preferable to randomization; if current results are similar, the less toxic arm might be preferred; if subset results are striking, only selected patients might be entered; or if results look generally poor on both arms, the investigators might use different treatments altogether. The consequences of this sort of informal study closure are inconclusive results and wasted resources. This can be avoided by not presenting interim results to investigators and having the necessary study monitoring performed by a data monitoring committee that has confidential access to results.

We have some evidence that informal and inappropriate stopping does occur when results are routinely reported, and that use of data monitoring committee minimizes such problems. Prior to 1985, SWOG trials were conducted without formal stopping guidelines or monitoring committees. Results of each ongoing trial were reported frequently, both at the semi-annual Group meetings and at national oncology meetings. Studies were closed by the vote of investigators active in the disease committee. We examined 14 of our trials conducted under these circumstances, and compared them to 14 trials matched on disease site from the North Central Cancer Treatment Group (NCCTG) which did have a monitoring committee policy (Green, Fleming, and O'Fallon, 1987). A variety of problems were discovered in the SWOG trials. Declining accrual occurred in five; two were inappropriately closed early; three studies were reported early as positive, but final results were not as convincing. Two trials did not even have set accrual goals. In contrast, NCCTG experienced minimal problems in the conduct of its trials. An accrual example from our investigation is shown in Table 3.1. SWOG accrual declined precipitously from 52 in the first 6-month interval to 16 in the final interval, due to what appeared to be convincing results. The study was closed early; after further follow-up results were no longer convincing. The matching study in NCCTG accrued steadily at about 20 per 6-month interval. Accrual on this study was completed and the final results were conclusive.

Of course we have to admit that since this comparison was not randomized, differences between the Groups other than monitoring committee approach could account for the problems noted in the SWOG studies. Still, the comparison is interesting.

Inappropriate early stopping from a statistical perspective is just one of the aspects of study monitoring. Safety monitoring is the most critical function of

TABLE 3.1

Accrual during Successive 6-Month Intervals for Two Trials

Interval	1	2	3	4	5	6	7	8
SWOG Trial	52	36	26	16				
NCCTG Trial	24	15	20	21	15	29	25	24

a monitoring committee. Deciding when there is sufficient evidence of harm to stop all or part of a trial can be especially difficult. It is at least reasonable to expect that a small group committed to careful review of all aspects of a trial will make better decisions than large groups acting informally based on impressions of the data. While there is general agreement that the primary responsibilities of a data monitoring committee are participant safety and study integrity, there is less agreement on the specific responsibilities. For instance, the majority of cancer cooperative groups agree that data monitoring committees don't review or approve the study design or evaluate the performance of individual study centers (George, 1993), but both of these functions were common in data monitoring committees of trials sponsored by the National Eye Institute (Hawkins, 1991). In some sense every aspect of study conduct affects safety and integrity. The number of oversight responsibilities assigned to a data monitoring committee will depend on what other resources and structures are available to the investigators (e.g., steering committee, operations office, statistical center, advisory board, sponsoring institution).

Even the specifics of the most basic task of the data monitoring committee, evaluation of interim results for evidence of benefit or harm, are not necessarily obvious. Questions (and our personal answers) include:

- How often should the data monitoring committee review interim data? (The answer to this should depend on how fast additional information becomes available on a trial. We generally recommend monitoring advanced disease studies, or any other study with rapidly accumulating events, every 6 months. Yearly monitoring may be sufficient for adjuvant or slowly accruing studies.)
- Should the primary outcome data be reviewed each time or should they be reviewed only at times of planned interim analyses? (All data should be available at every review, including primary outcome data, since the unexpected does occur.)
- Should treatment arms be blinded to the data monitoring committee or not? (Definitely not. If A looks better than B, the decision to continue could well be different if A is the control arm instead of the experimental arm.)
- Should a data monitoring committee decision that evidence is sufficient to close a trial be final, or should it be advisory only? (We would say advisory, but rarely overturned.)
- If advisory, advisory to whom—the funding agency? An executive group? The investigators? (Reports should go to the individuals with ultimate responsibility for the integrity of the trial.)
- Should a data monitoring committee be able to make major design changes to a trial? (No, the data monitoring committee may offer suggestions but design is the responsibility of the principal investigators. On the other hand, major design changes initiated by the principal investigators should be approved by the DMC.)

- Are data monitoring committee duties over when study accrual is complete, or should the data monitoring committee also decide when results are to be reported? (It should also decide when results are to be reported. There is often additional follow-up after the study is reported but this does not need a monitoring committee.)
- How much weight should be accorded to outside information versus current information on the study being monitored? (Definitive outside information cannot be ignored—but this begs the question of what is definitive. A single trial of moderate size probably is not definitive; two large trials probably are; a meta-analysis probably is not; see Chapter 9.)
- How much should results of secondary endpoints influence the decision to continue or not? (Not much unless toxic death is considered secondary.)
- How scary do results have to be to stop at a time other than a planned interim analysis? (Very scary, or the purpose of interim analyses is defeated.)
- When do accrual problems justify early closure? (When results won't be available until after they are no longer of interest.)
- Should confidential information ever be provided to other data monitoring committees or planning groups? (Sometimes. If study conduct will not be compromised by limited release of information, it might be reasonable to let investigators planning new trials know of potential problems or benefits to treatment arms they are considering. Risk to the ongoing trial includes leaked information or intelligent guesses as to the current status; risk to the new trial includes choosing an inappropriate arm based on early results that don't hold up.)

Every monitoring committee functions differently because no one has the same ethical, scientific, or practical perspectives. This means different committees might well come up with different answers to the same monitoring issues. To ensure some balance of opinions, it is best to have a variety of knowledgeable people as members of the committee.

3.7.1 Composition

We have suggested what is needed on a committee: variety, knowledge, balance of opinion. To ensure variety and knowledge, at least one person on the committee should: thoroughly understand the biologic rationale for the trial, know the clinical experience for the regimens being used, understand the statistical properties of the design, know the operational constraints on the trial, have a broad understanding of important questions and ongoing research in the disease being studied, have the study patients as major focus of concern. Extremes of opinion will unbalance a committee as a whole, and either lean it toward extreme decisions or make it impossible to reach decisions at all.

In particular, all members of a data monitoring committee must at least believe it is ethical to start accrual to the trial, and no one should be in a position of having a strong vested interest in the outcome.

"Vested interest" is a particularly troublesome concept. How it is defined and the degree to which it is tolerated has shifted significantly over time. Complete independence has been proposed as the only valid model for monitoring committees (Walters, 1993; Fleming, 1992). Independence means, in part, that no one on the committee has a major financial interest in the trial. We agree (although the definition of major is unclear). It is also construed to mean that no one has an academic interest in the trial either (for instance, an early report of a positive result could enhance a career or reputation). Here we are in less agreement. This interpretation of independence tends to bar from the committee those responsible for the science and the conduct of the trial, and this directly conflicts with the knowledge requirement. The people who know the most about the justification, background, conduct etc. of a trial are the ones running it. The next most knowledgeable people are the ones running similar trials, also viewed as a conflict. Finding thousands of knowledgeable people with no academic or financial conflicts for the hundreds of randomized cancer trials going on all the time is a daunting prospect.

Many also believe that no investigators who are entering patients on a trial should be on the data monitoring committee (DeMets et al., 1995). However, the case can be made that it is only such investigators who can really appreciate and grapple with the tension between the rights of patients on the trial and the benefits to future patients that might accrue (Harrington et al., 1994).

Certainly there are cases for which any appearance of possible conflict of interest would severely compromise a study. Highly visible or controversial trials and most industry trials must be protected from the appearance of bias or the results won't be accepted. Such trials will likely motivate data monitoring committee members to keep themselves well informed and to participate actively. On the other hand, low-profile and noncontroversial trials with only modest potential impact (many cancer treatment trials qualify) don't generate enough interest for appearance of conflict to be of great concern. They also don't generate enough interest to inspire independent monitors to spend a lot of time on them.

We now have had over 25 years experience with data monitoring committees in SWOG. In 1985 the group agreed that all Phase III studies should have monitoring committees and that explicit stopping/reporting guidelines should be included in all Phase III study designs. In the first DSMC model, committees consisted of the study statistician, the study coordinator, the study discipline coordinators if any, the disease committee chair, the group chair, the group statistician, a member of the group who was not directly involved in the study, and an NCI representative. Experience was positive, with few occurrences of the problems previously identified with group Phase III studies (Green and Crowley, 1993). Later modifications to this model included addition of representatives from other groups for intergroup trials, exclusion of drug company representatives ("The last priority [in the conduct of trials]

... is to make a profit and to pay dividends to shareholders." (Rockhold and Enas, 1993)) and specification of sanctions for premature disclosure of confidential results.

In response to political issues raised in AIDS trials (Ellenberg et al., 1992) and a high-profile incidence of fraud (Altaman, 1994; Goldberg and Goldberg, 1994; Christian et al., 1995), NCI mandated changes to Group monitoring committee structures to "ensure that DMCs for NCI sponsored Phase III therapeutic trials are operative, independent of trial investigators and clearly free of conflict of interest. Because clinical trials are under increasing public scrutiny, we must use procedures that protect our research against the appearance of impropriety. If we don't do this, then our excellent system for determining what treatments work and don't work may be threatened." (Simon and Ungerleider, 1992). Each group was instructed to create a single committee to oversee all Phase III trials coordinated by the group. Membership requirements were finalized after a number of adjustments to balance independence with knowledge. The majority of DSMC members now must be from outside of the group, including at least one outside patient advocate and at least one outside statistician. The group statistician and two NCI representatives are non-voting members. The group chair may not be a member. In addition to the DSMC each trial has a study committee charged with monitoring the study for toxicity, feasibility, and accrual.

This model does address concerns about potential scientific conflict of interest or misconduct by the Group leadership or by individual study chairs. With the creation of study committees, there is still ongoing careful monitoring for toxicity and procedural problems. We still have some concern, however, that a monitoring committee formulated this way does not have the time or sufficient knowledge about each individual study and its larger scientific context to be able to make adequately informed decisions on all 25+ studies being monitored. Furthermore, the information the committee receives comes from single individual involved in the trial (the study statistician) instead of from several knowledgeable about the conduct of the trial. Much as we would like to believe ourselves free of bias, the potential for conflict of interest (or even just mistakes) is clear.

3.7.2 Concluding Remarks on Monitoring Committees

Paul Meier (1975) has written that "although statistics has a role, the ethical problem of continuing or stopping an experiment is not primarily statistical. Neither is it especially a medical problem or a legal one. It is, in fact, a political problem, and I see no sensible way to cope with it outside a political framework." A few years ago we would have disagreed; now we are inclined to admit there is some truth to the contention. Still, we think there is room for a variety of models for monitoring committees to accommodate the political as well as the scientific and ethical issues. If we *start* with the assumption that most people will make judgments out of self-interest, no model at all will work.

3.8 Ethical Considerations

Ethical considerations for clinical trials center on the tension between care of individual patients and the need to study treatment effectiveness. The welfare of an individual patient should not be compromised by inclusion in a clinical trial. For instance, it may be perceived that assignment to standard treatment is not in the patient's best interest if standard treatment is not particularly effective. On the other hand, the welfare of patients in general requires clinical trials with control arms in order to identify those new treatments that are useful and discard those that are ineffective—in fact, treatment of patients with inadequately tested agents also raises ethical issues. There are too many examples of initially promising treatments shown in later trials to actually be detrimental to assume patient welfare is not being compromised when a new treatment is being used.

International guidance for ethics in medical research such as the Declaration of Helsinki (World Medical Association, 2004) emphasizes protection of health and rights of patients. Physicians' responsibilities to individual subjects are acknowledged:

- "Considerations related to the well-being of the human subject should take precedence over the interests of science and society."
- "It is the duty of the physician in medical research to protect the life, health, privacy, and dignity of the human subject."

    As are responsibilities to patients as a whole:
- "It is the duty of the physician to safeguard the health of the people."
- "Medical progress is based on research which ultimately must rest in part on experimentation involving human subjects."
- "The benefits, risks, burdens and effectiveness of a new method should be tested against those of the best current prophylactic, diagnostic, and therapeutic methods."

Guidance from the Declaration of Helsinki that helps inform decisions related to clinical trials include the requirement for careful assessment of risk-benefit (including a conclusion that risks can be adequately managed), agreement that the importance of the objective outweighs risks to individual patients, and a reasonable chance that future patients will benefit from the results. Severity of disease and availability of effective treatments are important considerations. Since cancer is usually life-threatening, observation only control arms are not appropriate if useful treatments are available.

Another key ethical principle is that of equipoise, i.e., the acknowledgement that usefulness of a new treatment is not yet known. Reasonable people may disagree as to when usefulness has been demonstrated, but as long as the general sense in the scientific community is one of uncertainty, comparative trials should be acceptable. Perhaps of equal or greater importance than demonstrating a treatment is effective, controlled trials may also demonstrate lack of effectiveness of purported breakthroughs. For instance, The Cardiac Arrhythmia Suppression Trial (Echt et al., 1991), noted in Chapter 1, demonstrated that encainide and flecainide increased the death rate in patients with recent myocardial infarction, despite convincing evidence of suppression of ventricular arrhythmia in previous studies. Many clinicians incorrectly believed the arrhythmia evidence made a control arm unethical. Fortunately, equipoise prevailed in the scientific community and allowed the trial to proceed, thereby sparing future patients a harmful treatment.

A particularly difficult circumstance for deciding whether a comparator arm is ethical is when a comparison involves injury or toxic effects to patients on an inactive treatment. In this case the benefits of a controlled trial may not be sufficient to proceed, although there are a number of examples of such trials. An example is a placebo controlled study of fetal nigral transplantation in Parkinson's disease (Olanow et al., 2003). Endpoints for this disease are subjective and placebo effects of treatment are likely, making blinding highly desirable. The sham surgery for this study consisted of placement of steriotactic frame, general anesthesia, scalp incision, partial burr hole, antibiotics, cyclosporin and PET studies, all of which are associated with risks to the patient. Discussion of the suitability of the design is presented by Freeman et al., 1999 and Macklin, 1999. As noted in the Freeman discussion, for a sham surgery to be considered the question should be important and not likely to become obsolete in the near future, the current state of evidence should be promising but inconclusive, there should be no satisfactory currently available treatments, intervention should be provided in addition to any standard therapy, and the question should not be answerable with less invasive designs. These criteria were met for the study. The ethical discussion in the two papers focuses on potential benefits to the placebo patients (including, for this trial, contribution to science, no cost standard medical treatment, later transplant at no cost if the procedure is found to be beneficial, spared other risks of transplant if found not beneficial) versus the risks (injury or death from sham procedure, inconvenience of a procedure with no potential clinical benefit except a placebo effect). Macklin concludes the sham surgery is not compatible with the principle of minimizing risk of harm and should not be done; Freeman et al. conclude the risks are reasonable with respect to possible benefits.

Another example of the issue of harm to patients on control treatment relates to regulatory requirements (Markman, 2010). The approved dose for pegilated liposomal doxorubicin (PLD) in ovarian cancer is 50 mg/m^2. Since this dose is associated with severe hand-foot syndrome (peeling, blisters, bleeding, hyperkeratosis, pain limiting self-care activities of daily living) in 25% of patients, the dose used in practice is usually 40 mg^2, which is associated with substantially less clinically relevant hand-foot syndrome. A review at a tertiary cancer center suggested that 96% of patients receive a dose of 40 mg or less, not 50. No Phase III trial of 40 versus 50 has been done, although other evidence suggests similar outcome for the two doses—e.g., similar results for two trials, one of PLD 40 versus gemcitabine and the other of PLD 50 versus gemcitabine (survival endpoint, similar gemcitabine regimens). The ethical issue is that for a new treatment to be approved it should be assessed against current approved standard treatment. Given the unacceptably severe side effects of 50 mg/m^2 and common use of 40 mg/m^2, Markman references the Nuremberg Code ("The experiment should be conducted as to avoid all unnecessary physical and mental suffering and injury.") and asks "Can the administration of PLD at a dose of 50 mg/m^2 to control patients participating in a randomized phase III trial possibly be considered to satisfy this rational ethical requirement?" Good question.

Another difficult circumstance occurs as evidence for or against a new treatment is accumulating. The most important function of a monitoring committee is protection of patients from harm—and it may also be the most difficult. How much evidence is required before it becomes unethical to treat with a possibly less effective or more toxic regimen? Much has been written on the subject (Byar et al., 1976; Gilbert et al., 1977; Mackillop and Johnston, 1986; Hellman and Hellman, 1991; Passamani, 1991; Piantadosi, 2005). These and other commentaries may make clear what some of the ethical questions are, but answers remain elusive. We offer two comments. First, there is no gold-standard statistical cutoff for a single endpoint that determines when results become convincing. Results of a study with 200 patients are not appreciably different when the last patient is omitted. A study with p-value 0.005 is barely more convincing than one with 0.0051. Stopping rules for a primary endpoint don't cover situations when unexpected or highly significant results emerge in secondary endpoints. The best statistics can do is provide guidelines that limit the number of mistaken conclusions from studies. Second, it is important to consider both responsibilities—the potential harm to patients on the study and potential harm to all future patients at risk for getting the treatments studied. The next patient on a trial with a trend is at risk for receiving the currently inferior arm. On the other hand, if the trend is false, it is not just the next patient registered at risk for the inferior arm, it is all future patients treated according to the published incorrect conclusion. The difficulty is particularly acute in oncology since relatively few new agents and regimens are found to be improvements—which means that a high percentage of early positive trends will, in fact, be false positives. Only additional accrual can clarify whether emerging differences are real or not.

Some investigators have tried to address ethical problems by requiring that the arm with the current best outcome be assigned to the next patient with higher probability than the other arms. This is called adaptive randomization or "play the winner"; see, for instance Wei and Durham (1978). There are a number of problems associated with use of these schemes. One is the possibility of too few patients being registered to one of the arms for a convincing result. A non-cancer example is a trial of extracorporeal membrane oxygenation (ECMO) versus control in newborns with severe respiratory failure (Bartlett et al., 1985). A Wei and Durham design was used, which resulted in the assignment of 9 patients to the experimental arm (all lived) and one to the control arm (who died). As discussed in Royall (1991), the trial generated criticism as being unconvincing because only a single patient received standard therapy. Interpretation of the trial depended on one's perception of the efficacy of standard treatment from historical information. Royall also discusses the ethics of the trial. The investigators were already convinced of the efficacy of ECMO; use of an adaptive allocation scheme was their solution to their ethical dilemma. Is it clear, however, that it is ethical to assign a smaller percent of patients to a treatment believed inferior when it is not ethical to assign 50%? In addition to ethical issues there are practical problems with this type of adaptive designs. Continuous updates and analysis may be difficult to accomplish, plus bias may result if time trends occur at the same time that percents registered to each arm are changing. Either of these could compromise the study. Further, any deviation from 1:1 randomization results in a loss of power, or an increase in sample size for a given power. For a recent discussion of these issues in the context of Bayesian adaptive randomization see Korn and Friedlin (2011) and accompanying editorial by Berry (2011).

Ethical issues will continue to be a challenge due to the inherent conflicts that arise between patient and societal best interest. In general, studies are considered ethical if the risk-benefit ratio is favorable, but magnitudes of risk and benefit are hard to quantify and reasonable people may disagree as to whether a particular study is acceptable.

3.9 Conclusion

We opened this chapter with a description of a dietary trial performed by the biblical Daniel. To conclude, let us see how Daniel's trial fared with respect to the design considerations discussed above. The objective is pretty clear: to compare two diets to decide which ones to feed the servants from the tribe of Judah. Eligibility is roughly described—youth (age not specified) who eat the king's food (how often and for how long not specified) and servants from the tribe of Judah. Treatment arms are specified, although not in detail—a meat and wine diet versus a vegetable and water diet. It is reasonable to assume there were no ethical issues. The endpoint is less satisfactory: "appearance" after 10 days is nonspecific, subjective, and does not adequately measure the long term health of the subjects. It is creditable that the endpoint was specified before the experiment was carried out, however. The treatment assignment is flawed. By assigning Daniel and his friends to the vegetable diet, the interpretation of the trial is compromised. Any difference in the two groups could be due to other cultural differences rather than diet. The magnitude of difference to be detected, assumptions used in sample size calculation and use of a monitoring committee are not specified in the biblical report; it is probably safe to assume these were not considered. So let us give Daniel 3.5/8—not bad for 2500 years ago.

4

Phase I and Phase I/II Trials

The trouble with people is not that they don't know but that they know so much that ain't so.

—Josh Billings (pseudonym for Henry Wheeler Shaw)

4.1 Phase I Trials

4.1.1 The Traditional 3 + 3 Design

The primary aim of a Phase I trial is to determine the maximum tolerated dose (MTD) of a new agent. These trials traditionally have been used for cytotoxic drugs, where it is assumed that higher doses will be more toxic, as well as more effective. For the determination of the MTD, the endpoint of interest is whether or not a patient experiences a dose limiting toxicity (DLT), where the definition of the type and level of toxicity considered dose limiting is stated in the protocol and determined by the disease and type of drug being tested. The subjects studied generally are patients with advanced disease for whom no effective standard therapy is available. A traditionally used design is a modified Fibonacci design. The sequence of dose levels used for escalation is often chosen to increase according to the following scheme: The second dose level is 2 times the first, the third is 1.67 times the second, the fourth is 1.5 times the third, the fifth is 1.4 times the fourth, and all subsequent doses are 1.33 times the previous. (The sequence is reminiscent of a Fibonacci sequence, which starts out with two numbers, after which each subsequent number is the sum of the two previous numbers. Fibonacci was a mathematician in Pisa who published and taught during the first half of the 13th century.)

Typically, three patients are entered at the first dose level, which is often chosen to be 10% of the mouse LD10 (dose at which 10% of mice die). If no patients experience a DLT, three patients are entered at the next dose level; if one patient experiences a DLT, three additional patients are treated at the same dose; if two or three patients experience DLTs, the dose is concluded to be above the MTD and dose escalation is discontinued. If six patients are treated, escalation continues if one patient experiences dose limiting toxicity,

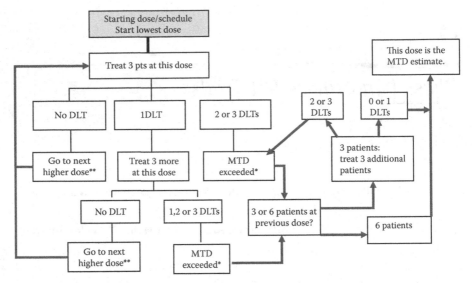

*If the MTD is exceeded at the lowest dose level stop. The MTD cannot be estimated.
** If there are no higher dose levels, stop. The MTD cannot be estimated.

FIGURE 4.1
Schema for traditional Phase I design.

otherwise the dose is concluded to be above the MTD and escalation ends. When a dose is concluded to be above the MTD the next lower dose is declared the MTD, if six patients have already been treated at that dose. Otherwise three additional patients are treated at the next lower dose, and if zero or one have DLTs this is declared the MTD. If two or more have DLTs there is further de-escalation according to the same scheme. The design continues until the MTD is declared or until the first dose is concluded to be above the MTD (Figure 4.1).

Although the traditional design is useful, it is not optimal in any sense. This design does not converge to the true MTD, confidence intervals perform poorly (nominal 80% confidence intervals do not include the correct value 80% of the time, 95% intervals are often of infinite length), and it is sensitive to both the starting dose and the dose-toxicity relationship (Storer, 1989). The traditional design always targets the dose at which 1/6–1/3 of patients experience severe toxicity. This is not always a suitable choice and there is no straightforward way to adapt this design for different criteria. Furthermore, with the traditional design too many patients may be treated at low doses. Since the usual assumption justifying Phase I designs is that both toxicity and effectiveness are increasing functions of increasing dose, implying that the MTD is also the most effective dose, ethical issues are raised. Patients volunteer for Phase I studies, in part, as a final hope of benefit, so to the extent possible potentially efficacious doses should be used. As an example of how the traditional Phase I may not work well, consider an agent with modest increases in toxicity for lower doses followed by a steep rise for higher doses.

Dose	0.05	0.1	1.6	2.4	3.2	4.3	5.7
True % of patients with DLT	4%	6%	9%	13%	22%	40%	60%

With this dose, DLT relationship the expected number of patients tested at inadequate doses of 1.6 or less is approximately 11. On the other hand, the chance of testing the highly toxic 5.7 dose is 15%. In addition, the median dose chosen is 2.4 instead of the correct dose of 3.2. Too many patients are treated at both high and low doses, plus the wrong dose is chosen as the MTD, illustrating the need for improvement in Phase I design.

4.1.2 Improving Phase I Designs

Alternatives to the traditional design have been investigated to decrease the number of patients treated at low doses and to improve the MTD estimate. Although the small sample sizes at each dose for most Phase I studies preclude very good statistical properties, newer designs may perform better than the traditional design.

In order to assess the performance of Phase I designs, an explicit definition of the MTD is required. The general idea in a Phase I trial is to find a dose to recommend for Phase II testing that does not result in too many patients experiencing a dose limiting toxicity, with "not too many" often approximately 1/3. Mathematically, if $\Psi(d)$ is the function representing the probability of DLT at dose d, then the MTD is the dose d_{MTD} that satisfies $\Psi(d_{MTD}) = 1/3$ (Figure 4.2). We will use 0.33 as the target probability of DLT throughout the rest of the chapter, but note another value might be a more appropriate choice for a particular study.

The following are various possible ways to approach improvement in Phase I design.

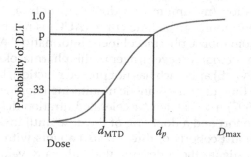

FIGURE 4.2
Dose–toxicity curve. The MTD in this example is the dose at which the probability of DLT = 0.33.

4.1.2.1 Start at a Higher Dose?

Horstmann et al., 2005 reported on 460 Phase I trials in adults sponsored by the Cancer Therapy Evaluation Program of the National Cancer Institute between 1991 and 2002. The overall toxic death rate for these trials was 0.49% and grade 4 events were reported in 14.3% of patients for whom this information was available. Of note, responses (CR or PR) were observed in 10.6%, with stability observed in 34.1%. Response varied by type of trial; for instance, single agent chemotherapy trials had fewer responses, but more stable disease than multi-agent chemotherapy trials. These observations might suggest that the Phase I trials generally have a reasonable risk-benefit profile, with possible room for a modestly more aggressive approach.

Starting with 10% of mouse LD10 (.1MLD10) often results in many dose escalations before the MTD is reached, so some savings would be possible if starting with higher doses could be assumed sufficiently safe. This possibility was discussed in a review article by Eisenhauer et al. (2000). For 14 agents with detailed information available in 21 trials, .1MLD10 was safe in all 14, .2LD10 was safe in 12, and .3MLD10 was safe for 8. "Unsafe" for this examination was defined as three or fewer dose levels required to reach the MTD. Considered in a different way, among 57 new agents from the literature, in all but one the MTD was equal to or greater than .1MLD10 and the median first toxic dose was eight times .1MLD10. The authors concluded that although .2MLD10 might be suitable in certain cases with no interspecies differences in toxicology, the recent adoption of more aggressive escalation strategies means that a change would result in minimal efficiency gain.

A setting in which higher starting doses is usually reasonable is that of new combinations for agents with Phase I testing already done. In this case starting doses moderately below the single agent MTD are employed unless significant drug interactions are considered possible.

4.1.2.2 Modify the Traditional Algorithm?

Various proposals to speed up the Phase I process involve fewer patients and larger dose increases early on, followed by more conservative escalations and more patients when targets are neared. Collins et al. (1986, 1990) proposed accelerated escalation (maximum of a doubling) until a target area under the plasma concentration versus time curve (AUC) is reached, with the target determined from mouse pharmacokinetic information. Although savings were noted in Phase I trials of several agents, this pharmacokinetically guided dose escalation (PGDE) approach has not proven practical, largely due to the drawback of real-time pharmacokinetic monitoring (Collins, 2000).

Simon et al. (1997) investigated "accelerated titration designs," involving one patient per cohort and a doubling of the dose until toxicity is observed, followed by standard cohorts of three to six patients with smaller dose increments. To investigate these designs the authors developed 20 different dose-toxicity models based on results from 20 real studies, and assessed how well 4 different Phase I strategies performed for each model. Design 1 was the

TABLE 4.1

Accelerated Titration Designs

	Standard	Accelerated	Accelerated	Accelerated
Design	1	2	3	4
Dose increase	×1.4	×1.4	×1.96	×1.96
Cohort size	3, 6	1	1	1
Rule to switch to standard		DLT cycle 1 or 2nd grade 2 cycle 1	DLT cycle 1 or 2nd grade 2 cycle 1	1st DLT or 2nd grade 2 any cycle
Intra-patient escalation	No	Yes	Yes	Yes

traditional design with dose increases of 40%; Design 2 had cohort size one with 40% dose increases until a DLT or two grade 2 toxicities were observed in cycle one, at which point the design switched to the traditional approach; Design 3 was the same as Design 2 except increases until the switch were 96%; Design 4 switched when DLTs or two grade 2s were observed in any cycle. Design 1 did not include intra-patient dose escalation while Designs 2, 3, and 4 did (Table 4.1).

The four designs were assessed through simulation using the 20 models. For those unfamiliar with simulations, these are experiments done on the computer. A set of random numbers is generated by the computer and transformed into outcomes for a "study," such as toxicity grades for Phase I studies, response for Phase II or survival and censoring times for Phase III. The transformations are chosen so that the results have a particular distribution (in this case the distributions correspond to the expected toxicity grades for each of the models, for survival the distribution is often the exponential distribution discussed in Chapter 2). More sets of random numbers are then generated to create more "studies." Each of these "studies" can be analyzed and analysis results summarized in tables. The summaries allow us to assess the methods of analysis we use. For instance, in theory, 0.05 level tests erroneously reject the null hypothesis of no difference in exactly 5% of studies for which there are, in fact, no differences, but in practice this is just an approximation. Generating hundreds of studies allows us to see how good the approximations actually are under specific conditions. For Phase I we can assess how often a particular Phase I design arrives at the proper dose under various assumptions.

One must keep in mind that the results from this investigation are based on models of 20 trials of chemotherapeutic agents, so may not reflect the whole range of Phase I trials. Results would differ for different model assumptions and different types of agents. Note also that dose doubling in a first-in-human trial might entail too much risk. Nevertheless, simulation results from the paper suggest savings in sample size using the accelerated titration approach with only modest increases in grade 3–4 toxicity (Table 4.2). In addition, although all designs pick the true MTD with the highest frequency, Design 1 has the highest frequency of MTD estimates below the correct value, while Design 3 has the lowest. The authors emphasize the need for careful

TABLE 4.2

Simulation Results for Accelerated Titration Designs 1–4

Design	1	2	3	4
Average N	39.9	24.4	20.7	21.2
# trials with average N >50 (of 20 trials)	6	0	0	0
Average # patients with worst grade toxicity = 0 or 1	23.3	7.9	3.9	4.8
Without intra-patient escalation		10.5	6.5	7.0
Average # patients with worst grade toxicity = 3 or 4	7.4	9.2	11.1	9.4
Without intra-patient escalation		7.4	8.9	8.2

definitions of dose limiting toxicity and of the toxicity level considered sufficiently low for intra-patient escalation.

Experience with accelerated titration designs has accumulated since the original publication. Heath et al. (2009) reported on nine Phase 1 chemotherapy trials done at Wayne State University and published between 1995 and 2005. Four of these were conducted according to the traditional design and five with accelerated titration designs. The average number of patients treated on the traditionally designed trials was 34 versus an average of 23.8 patients on the accelerated titration trials. The average number of dose levels was 8.8 (range 7–11) for traditional and 10.6 (range 7–15) for accelerated titration. Average study duration (25–26 months) was similar for the two designs. Penel et al. (2009) compared the performance of these two types of designs in 270 recently (1997–2008) published Phase I trials. Accelerated titration had been used in 10% of these. For this data set the average number of patients on the accelerated titration trials was not reduced compared to traditional design. The average number of dose levels assessed was significantly higher for accelerated titration than for traditional (7 versus 5), and the proportion of patients treated at doses below phase 2 recommended dose was significantly lower (46% versus 56%). As for the Wayne State trials, the study duration was not shorter. In practice it appears there is some advantage to accelerated titration designs, although improvement is modest. While it is promising that a larger number of dose levels was examined and that fewer patients were treated at inadequate dose levels, the hoped for improvement in duration was not observed.

Storer (1989, 2011) also developed a design that initially adds and evaluates one patient at a time. Storer further modified the traditional design by allowing more flexibility in escalation and de-escalation ("up and down design"). If the first patient does not have a DLT, the dose is escalated in single patients until a DLT is observed; if the first patient does have a DLT, the dose is de-escalated in single patients until no DLT is observed. At this point accrual to dose levels is done in threes, with dose level increased if no DLTs are observed, not changed if one is observed, and decreased if two or three are observed. The study ends after a fixed number of cohorts of patients has been accrued. At the conclusion of accrual the MTD is estimated from a logistic model. As for the accelerated titration design, simulations have shown that this procedure has better properties compared to the traditional design, including improved MTD estimates and fewer patients treated at low dose levels without greatly increasing the proportion of patients treated at unacceptably high doses. Ivanova et al. (2003) investigated a number of up and down designs and noted that using accumulated information to inform the choice of dose in the next patient was better than the use of just the results from the most recent trial patient.

4.1.2.3 Use Model-Based Designs?

The algorithmic approaches of the traditional Phase I or up and down designs lack flexibility in choice of target probability of DLT. Continual reassessment methodology (CRM) is a different approach to improving Phase I designs that allows specification of any target probability. CRM designs use model-based criteria for dose escalation in addition to a model-based estimate of the MTD. The original proposal for these designs (O'Quigley et al., 1990) is to recalculate an estimate of the MTD after each patient is treated and assessed for toxicity, and then to treat the next patient at the dose level closest to this estimate. The final estimate of the MTD occurs after a prespecified number of patients have been treated. The most attractive aspects of this type of design are that all previous results are used which, as noted above, improves design performance over the traditional design and the potential for more efficiently arriving at an MTD estimate. See Figure 4.3 for an illustration of the hoped for improvement due to use of a CRM design.

Despite the potential of the original CRM design, concerns were expressed. Because CRM designs use a statistical model based on a priori assumptions about the dose-toxicity relationship to select the starting dose, it is possible that the first dose used is not the lowest dose thought to be clinically reasonable. Of additional concern, these designs may result in dose escalations that skip several dose levels, in treatment of only one patient at a dose level

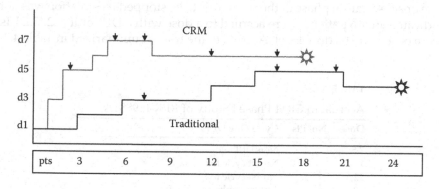

FIGURE 4.3
Potential benefits of CRM design: Fewer total number of patients, fewer patients treated at low doses.

when patient heterogeneity is high and time delays in waiting for toxicity assessment after each patient (a problem shared with the initial stage of the Storer and accelerated titration designs). Various modifications of the basic CRM design have been proposed to address these issues, such as starting at the first dose regardless of the initial estimate, not restricting to one patient at each stage and not allowing dose levels to be skipped (Goodman et al., 1995); using an initial stage similar to Storer or accelerated titration (successively higher doses given to one or two patients until toxicity is observed) to target the appropriate dose range before switching to CRM (Moeller, 1995); or requiring that the closest dose below the current estimate be used instead of the closest dose. Some efficiency is lost with such modifications, but safety is usually the greater consideration. Another adaptation concerns when to stop the trial. Rather than stopping after a fixed number of patients, it may be reasonable to specify a rule to allow early stopping if the MTD is settled before the maximum sample size (e.g., if N subjects are treated at the same dose). Also see O'Quigley (2011).

An interesting CRM variation is the LMH-CRM design due to Huang and Chappell (2008). They propose treating cohorts of three at each CRM stage, but to treat each patient at three different doses (low, medium, and high, with some restrictions on how many dose levels can be skipped). This approach has potential to provide better final estimates of the MTD as well as to limit the number of patients treated at low doses.

A Phase I study of RPR 109881A provides an example of a CRM design used in practice (Gelmon et al., 2000). Dose levels of 7.5, 15, 22.5, 30, 37.5, 45, 52.5, 60, and 67.5 were chosen for study and the target DLT probability was specified at 0.5. The MTD was estimated to be 45 prior to the start of the trial and the starting dose was chosen to be 7.5 based on a prior estimate of 5% chance of DLT at this dose. CRM modifications used included at least one patient per dose level, increases of at most one dose level, no increase over the current MTD estimate, at least three patients prior to escalation if a non-DLT is observed, and at least six patients at a dose level with one DLT. The dose escalation phase of the study was to be stopped if escalation was not indicated after 6 patients were accrued to a dose with a DLT or if $\geq 2/3$ DLTs were observed at a dose level. Accrual to the trial is summarized in Table 4.3.

TABLE 4.3

Accrual to CRM Phase I Study of RPR 109881A

Dose	No. Pts	Cycle One DLTs
7.5	4	Non-DLT
15	1	No 1st cycle tox
22.5	1	No 1st cycle tox
30	2	1 pt had only a single dose
37.5	3	Non-DLT
45	12	Expanded to 12
52.5	6	Unable to increase dose after 6 pts (3 DLTs)

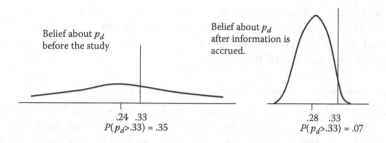

Belief about p_d before the study

Belief about p_d after information is accrued.

.24 .33
$P(p_d > .33) = .35$

.28 .33
$P(p_d > .33) = .07$

FIGURE 4.4
Illustration of Bayesian characterization of belief about parameter p_d before study start and after information is accrued.

The design worked well, in part due to the good initial guess concerning MTD. Two cohorts needed only one patient, so the trial resulted in a modest reduction in patients needed. Few patients were treated at the lowest doses and reasonable decisions were made.

Another approach to Phase I design, related to CRM, is the Escalation with Overdose Control (EWOC) design (Babb et al., 1998; Tighiouart et al., 2005). Instead of considering only the MTD, the probabilities of DLT for all doses are considered in EWOC designs, with the aim of restricting the probability of overdosing.

Both CRM and EWOC designs use Bayesian methods; EWOC provides an illustration of how these methods are used. One of the features of Bayesian methods is that parameters are assigned distributions that reflect uncertainty about the value of the parameter. There is significant uncertainty before a Phase I study is done, so typically a distribution with large variance is assigned. As information is accrued, the distribution is updated to reflect more certainty about the value of the parameter (Figure 4.4). In the EWOC setting the parameters of interest are the probabilities of DLT for each dose d, denoted p_d. Patients are not treated with dose d if the chance (according to current belief) that d is greater than the MTD is too high (i.e., an unacceptable chance that p_d is greater than 0.33). A typical choice for unacceptable might be greater than 25%, with 25% or lower acceptable. Figure 4.4 also illustrates when doses would be acceptable. For the curve on the left the estimated probability of DLT is 0.24, which is below the target of 0.33, but there is a 35% chance that it is actually greater than 0.33 so the dose would not be used. For the curve on the right, the estimated probability is higher at 0.28, but the chance of being over 0.33 is only 7%, so in this case the dose could be used. For the EWOC approach the highest dose for which the estimated chance of overdose is 25% or less is assigned to the next patient.

EWOC designs do indeed reduce overdosing compared to CRM, but the price paid is longer trial time. Chu et al., 2009, combined the EWOC and CRM approaches into a hybrid design involving an increase in the acceptable chance from conservative early on (10%) to more liberal later (50%) allowing the CRM approach to be used later on in the study after toxicity is better characterized. This approach is a compromise between efficiency and safety, as it tends to reach a conclusion sooner than EWOC while resulting in fewer overdosed patients than CRM.

4.1.2.4 Alternative Approaches for Biologic Agents?

For agents with low toxicity potential and with specified biologic targets, the standard assumptions justifying Phase I designs may not apply. As noted above, a Phase I design for a cytotoxic cancer agent generally has the objective of identifying the MTD. Since it is assumed that higher doses will be both more toxic and more effective against the cancer, toxicity is the only primary endpoint. For a biologic agent, on the other hand, the toxicity-dose curve may be quite shallow and the assumption of increasing response with increasing dose may not be correct; responses may plateau instead of increasing at high doses. The Phase I objective for this type of agent might more suitably be to identify doses that produce an acceptable level of biologic response subject to acceptable toxicity.

CRM approaches could be used in this setting as well as the chemotherapy setting. Hunsberger et al. (2005) took a different approach and proposed easily implemented designs for targeted agents when toxicity can reasonably be assumed minimal over a wide range of doses. (If minimal toxicity is not anticipated, joint assessment of toxicity and biologic response as discussed in the next section of this chapter may be appropriate.) Dose escalation is based on patient response, defined as occurrence of the desired effect on the target. A potentially useful approach is to consider the slope of the line describing response rate as a function of dose. The slope is estimated from the highest 4 doses, with cohorts of 3 patients per dose. Escalation stops when the slope is estimated to be 0 or less (i.e., the response rate is not increasing) and the dose with the highest response rate is chosen for further testing. The goal is not necessarily to reach a dose with maximum response (which could require an extended trial with a large sample size), but rather a dose within 10% of the maximum in the dose-response plateau. Simulations suggest that this design is promising when there aren't too many dose levels before response plateaus.

Of course new biologic agents often do not yet have a molecularly targeted endpoint that can be assumed related to clinical outcome. Another challenge is that biologic response (such as immune response) can take several months to develop, and that it is patients with normal biologic function who might be expected to have reasonable responses to biologic agents. Thus, in addition to considering alternative designs, alternative eligibility criteria might also need to be considered since the typical Phase I population, with short-term survival and compromised function, may not be suitable.

4.1.3 Phase I Conclusion

Compromise on design characteristics is a necessity when choosing a Phase I design. Different methods provide advantages with respect to various factors such as number of patients needed, accuracy of estimates, minimization of number treated with doses above the MTD, minimization of number treated with ineffective doses or number of doses sampled. Not all factors can be optimized, so study-specific needs must be carefully considered. This often involves assessing candidate designs using simulation under various dose-toxicity relationships considered plausible for the agent to be studied.

It is clear that we can improve on the standard Phase I design. Various new designs have been implemented in practice (see Berlin et al., 1998, for an example of a Storer design, Dees et al., 2000, for an example of a PGDE design, Sessa et al., 2000, for an example of an accelerated titration, Gelmon et al., 2000 for a CRM design). Accelerated titration and CRM variations have gained in acceptance, but the modified Fibonacci, three-patient-per-dose-level approach still remains the most common approach. Penel et al., 2009, noted that of the 288 Phase I dose seeking trials of systemic therapy reviewed, 243 used the standard design. Consensus on the best Phase I strategies among the various available alternative designs has yet to develop.

4.2 Phase I/II Designs

4.2.1 Combining Phase I and Phase II

Occasionally the patients treated at the MTD of a Phase I design are included as part of a subsequent Phase II study. The approach of conducting two studies under one protocol with a limited number of patients included in each study may seem efficient, but the goals of Phase I studies and Phase II studies of efficacy are often different enough that a combined protocol may not be sensible. If the Phase I is a typical all solid tumor trial, very few patients will be eligible for a disease specific Phase II. Even if several are eligible, note that patients chosen as suitable for experimentation with possibly ineffective or toxic doses of an agent are systematically different from those chosen as suitable to test for activity of the agent, possibly biasing the Phase II results. Further, the last several patients on a Phase I study, by design, have experienced a certain level of toxicity. If toxicity and antitumor activity are related in any way, then use of patients from the dose-finding part of a trial as part of an efficacy assessment may also bias the results. Consideration of operational difficulty in conducting two studies within one protocol is also a factor. Generally it is preferred that new patients be used for the Phase II. In any case, two sequential studies with different objectives and different endpoints, do not constitute a formal Phase I/II study design.

Related to this is the practice of adding an expansion cohort in a specified population after the MTD is declared in order to further characterize toxicity and to examine for early signals of activity. Criteria for changing the recommended Phase II dose or deciding not to pursue a Phase II based on efficacy outcomes are rarely provided. Because the $3 + 3$ design requires <33% of patients to have DLTs, it is often assumed that observation of <33% DLTs is also a suitable rule for the expansion cohort, but this is not necessarily a reasonable criterion. For instance, the MTD at the end of a Phase I trial typically will have 1/6 patients with DLT. The 90% confidence interval for this is from 0.01 to 0.58, leaving open the possibility of significant toxicity at the chosen dose. If the 33% rule is applied to 10 patients in an expansion cohort then 3/10 would be acceptable—but the 90% confidence interval for 3/10 is from 0.08 to 0.61, which provides no better assurance of safety than 1/6. If the MTD cohort and expansion cohort are considered jointly, 5/16 would be acceptable, but the upper bound of the confidence interval for this is 0.55, still providing limited assurance. It is also typical to examine an expansion cohort for response to treatment. If there is no signal a Phase II might not be pursued. This is also problematic, unless the expansion cohort is properly sized. The 90% confidence interval for 0/10 is from 0 to 0.26, which does not provide assurance that the agent is inactive. An efficacy decision based on an expansion cohort amounts to a small, informal first stage of a Phase II without the appropriate adjustments for an initial test. If an expansion cohort is planned, as is frequently the case now in tumor-specific trials of a new agent in combination, criteria for decisions based on the cohort should be detailed. As an example, Hoering et al. (2011) suggest investigating several doses at or below the estimated MTD, with a formal pick the winner design based on toxicity and response to choose the final dose for further Phase II testing.

4.2.2 Phase I/II

A formal phase I/II design is a design that jointly assesses toxicity and efficacy at various dose levels in order to choose a dose with an acceptable risk-benefit profile for further study. The initial publication in the Phase I/II area (Gooley et al., 1994) examined a number of ad hoc up-down designs with the dose for the next cohort based on the number of patients in the current cohort without efficacy (rejection after transplant) or with toxicity (graft versus host disease), and identified one with reasonable properties. The major contribution of this paper was use of simulation as a tool to calibrate parameters in order to achieve acceptable design characteristics, an approach now routinely used. Various other designs are now available, both for two binary outcomes (efficacy and toxicity) and for a three-level outcome (efficacy and no toxicity, no efficacy and no toxicity, toxicity).

O'Quigley et al. (2001) generalized continual reassessment methods (CRM) to address the three-outcome case. The motivating example was an HIV application. For each patient failure occurs either if there is unacceptable toxicity or toxicity is acceptable but viral load is not reduced, while success is defined as acceptable toxicity and reduced viral load. A true probability of success of p_0 is specified as unsatisfactory and p_1 is specified as promising. For this approach to design it is assumed that toxicity increases as a function of dose and that efficacy given no toxicity also increases as a function of dose. (Note: The former is usually a reasonable assumption, the latter may not be.) The probability of success is a function of these two increasing functions and will not itself be an increasing function of dose. CRM methods for toxicity are used initially, but then as success information is accumulated for a particular dose, tests of p_0 versus p_1 are done. Concluding in favor of p_1 stops the trial with a recommendation of further study of that dose. Concluding in favor of p_0 leads to the conclusion that the dose and all lower doses should not be considered for further study. Simulations suggest that the procedure does well so long as doses with poorly distinguishable toxicity levels have distinct efficacy differences.

A proposal by Thall and Cook (2004) accommodates both the two binomial endpoint case and the three outcome case and also allows for a nonincreasing dose-efficacy relationship. Key to this approach is specification of efficacy-toxicity trade-off contours. For the two outcome case, information elicited from investigators includes the minimum acceptable probability of efficacy (E_{min}, occurring when there is no toxicity), the maximum acceptable probability of toxicity (T_{max}, occurring when there is 100% efficacy), and a third pair of equally desirable probabilities intermediate between the extremes (E_c, T_c). These three points are used to construct a set of efficacy-toxicity trade-off contours (Figure 4.5). The basic outline of the procedure is to treat the first cohort at the starting dose specified by the physician. For each cohort after the first, the set of acceptable doses given the current data is calculated. A dose x is acceptable if it is reasonably likely (according to current belief as quantified by the Bayesian distribution) that the efficacy probability is larger than E_{min} and that it is reasonably likely that the toxicity probability is less than T_{max}. If there are no acceptable doses then trial is closed and no dose is selected. If there are acceptable doses, the next cohort is treated either at the next untried dose level or at the most desirable level, whichever is lower. The most

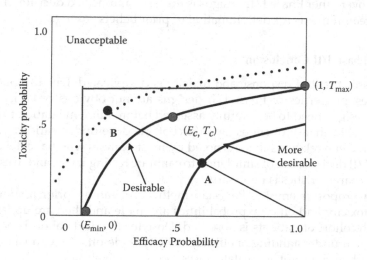

FIGURE 4.5
Efficacy-toxicity trade-off contours.

desirable dose level is the one on the most desirable contour (also illustrated in Figure 4.5). If the trial is not stopped early and there are acceptable doses remaining at the end of the trial then the most desirable of the remaining doses is chosen for further study. For an example of a Thall and Cook design, see Thall et al. (2006). Simulations suggest the approach is promising. Bekele and Shen (2005) address the case of binary toxicity and continuous efficacy, such as a biomarker expression outcome, also with promising results.

Zhang et al. (2006) addressed the three outcome case with a proposed Bayesian "TriCRM" design potentially useful for joint assessment of toxicity and efficacy for biologic agents. The motivating example here is an agent that boosts hemoglobin (Hb) in patients with Hb below the normal range. The three outcomes are no response (Hb remains below the normal range), response (Hb in the normal range), and toxicity (Hb above the normal range). Toxicity is assumed to increase with dose, no response is assumed to decrease with dose, and response need not have a straightforward relationship with dose. Models are used to describe the dose-outcome relationship. If there is toxicity other than high Hb, outcome is classified as toxicity. After a cohort of patients is assessed, Bayesian estimates of probability of toxicity for each dose, $p_t(d)$, and probability of response for each dose, $p_r(d)$, are updated. Doses considered for the next cohort are those for which current $p_t(d)$ estimates are below a specified threshold. The dose chosen for the next cohort is the one that maximizes $p_r(d) - \lambda p_t(d)$. If λ is 0, this is just the dose with the highest response estimate subject to an acceptable toxicity. If λ is > 0 then there is a penalty for higher levels of toxicity. At the end of the trial the same decision rule is applied and the chosen dose is termed the biologically optimal dose (BOD). Simulations were done and, as for the other methods described in this section, properties were promising. An advantage to this design over other Phase I/II designs is the less complicated decision rule and fewer requirements for determination of prior beliefs.

4.2.3 Phase I/II Conclusion

Joint assessment of response and toxicity is complicated. Due to small sample sizes, properties of Phase I/II designs are not obvious or easily calculated. Designs need to be carefully assessed before implementation to assure a reasonable chance of choosing an acceptable dose under various possible dose-outcome relationships. As noted by most authors who have developed Phase I/II designs, use of simulation to calibrate testing levels and to estimate design characteristics is necessary.

Most proposals employ Bayesian methods, meaning prior assumptions about toxicity and efficacy probabilities are made and then are updated after each cohort of patients is observed. Dose for the next cohort is based on the current understanding of efficacy-toxicity trade-offs. Care must be taken with such designs not to escalate doses too aggressively since early estimates based on uncertain assumptions may be misleading. An additional issue for Bayesian approaches is that identification of the next dose is not a matter of counting the number of dose limiting toxicities; instead it requires significant computation to update the distributions of the parameters in order to identify the most likely useful dose. Yet another issue is the effort it takes to design the studies. Extensive discussions concerning design parameters are needed followed by the necessary simulations. It may take several iterations to identify an appropriate design.

The main advantage to a Phase I/II design is specification of the now informal criteria used for efficacy assessment on Phase I. However, considering the labor intensity of designing Phase I/II trials, the likely difficulties with implementation, and the likely delays in waiting for efficacy information before the next dose level can be decided, these designs would not generally be recommended for routine use. An area where Phase I/II designs might be worth the extra complications may be in proof of concept assessment. For example, a joint assessment of toxicity and immune response for an immunologic agent could provide valuable information. For this type of setting Phase I/II approaches could potentially lead to better choices of dose for further development than approaches considering only toxicity, especially in cases where the dose-toxicity relationship is not strong.

5

Phase II Trials

Baseball is the only field of endeavor where a man can succeed 3 times out of 10 and be considered a success.

—Ted Williams

Phase II trials provide the testing ground for the development of definitive Phase III trials through the screening of new agents for antitumor activity, and by piloting new treatment combinations and schedules. In recent years the focus of Phase II trial design has undergone a substantial shift in emphasis, partially in response to the development of targeted agents, and in part on the popularity of randomized Phase II designs.

No matter what the design, the essential elements of Phase II designs include a limited sample size, compromises in Types I and II error, and a recognition that definitive clinical conclusions are not to be drawn from these exploratory trials.

We begin first with a discussion of traditional Phase II designs.

5.1 Single-Arm Phase II Designs

Standard Phase II studies of investigational new drugs (INDs) are used to screen new agents for antitumor activity and to decide which agents should be tested further. Traditionally, these designs have most typically been single-arm studies using short-term endpoints (usually tumor response in cancer studies) in limited numbers of patients. The statistical underpinning of a single-arm design can be formulated as a test of the null hypothesis $H_0 : p = p_0$ versus the alternative hypothesis $H_1 : p = p_1$, where p is the probability of the primary outcome (e.g., response), p_0 is the probability which, if true, would mean that the agent was not worth studying further, and p_1 is the probability which, if true, would mean it would be important to identify the agent as active and to continue studying it. (See Chapter 2 for a discussion of hypothesis testing.) Typically, p_0 is chosen to be a value at or somewhat below the historical probability of response to standard treatment for the same stage of disease, and p_1 is sufficiently higher, selected to identify a clinically meaningful improvement over the historical value. The choices of

p_0 and p_1 are dependent on definitions of outcome, patient selection factors, and regimen characteristics. The most relevant historical experience is from the same group of investigators planning the current trial. Phase II studies done at single institutions often include better risk patients, more consistent treatment delivery and more liberal response definitions than studies done in the Cooperative Groups; thus single institution studies tend to provide poor estimates upon which to base choices of p_0 and p_1 for a multicenter study.

Both the choice of endpoint and the specification of null and alternative hypotheses require careful thought in the design of Phase II trials. Historically, tumor shrinkage (response) was the norm when most Phase II trials tested cytotoxic agents. As single agents, newer targeted therapies often have little impact on tumor shrinkage, and their main effect appears to be in tumor stabilization, resulting in longer progression-free survival (PFS) or overall survival (OS). Thus, an alternative endpoint such as 6-month survival may be appropriate.

The choice of null and alternative hypotheses should be based on current experience, particularly if a review of prior Phase II results suggests changes over time. As definitions and treatments change, the old historical estimates of these probabilities may not remain applicable. For example, in the 1990s the median survival for patients with advanced/metastatic colorectal cancer was approximately 12 months, whereas it is now nearly double.

5.1.1 The Standard SWOG Phase II Design

Our standard approach to the design of Phase II IND trials (Green and Dahlberg, 1992) is to accrue patients in 2 stages, with significance level (probability of rejecting $H_0 : p = p_0$ when it is true) approximately 0.05 and power (probability of accepting $H_1 : p = p_1$ when it is true) approximately 0.9. A specified number of patients is targeted for a first stage of accrual, and when that target is approached the study is closed temporarily while responses are assessed. We stop the study early if the agent appears unpromising— specifically, if the alternative hypothesis is rejected at the 0.02 level after the first stage of accrual. If the study is not stopped early, it is reopened to a second stage of accrual. We conclude the agent is promising only if H_0 is rejected after the second stage of accrual.

SWOG S0415, a trial of cetuximab as second-line therapy in patients with metastatic esophageal cancer (Gold et al., 2010), provides an example of the SWOG Phase II design. This trial was designed to evaluate overall survival at 6 months. The null hypothesis was specified as $H_0 : p_0 = 0.3$ and the alternative $H_1 : p_1 = 0.5$. The standard design in this case is to accrue 30 patients initially, with 25 more patients if 9 or more patients survive for at least 6 months in the first 30, and to conclude that the regimen is worth pursuing if at least 23 patients of 55 survive for at least 6 months. Note that 23/55 or 0.42 is not the alternative $p_1 = 0.5$. Rather, it is the lowest observed 6-month OS probability that leads to a decision in favor of the alternative true probability of 0.5 as opposed to the null hypothesized probability of 0.3.

There are numerous designs for the conduct of single-arm Phase II trials (others will be described later). Our approach to the design of Phase II trials has evolved in response to various practical considerations.

First, for ethical reasons it is important to be able to stop subjecting patients to new agents as soon as we have convincing evidence the agent is ineffective. For example, suppose in the S0415 trial that there are only 3 patients who survived past 6 months in the first 10 patients. The treatment isn't looking as if it is benefiting patients—should the trial be stopped? The statistical problem here is judging whether or not this is convincing evidence of ineffectiveness. In this example, 7 failures is probably not convincing. For instance, if the new agent actually has a 50% chance of surviving past 6 months, groups of 10 patients would ON AVERAGE have 5 patients survive, but in about 17% of groups of 10 there would be 3 or fewer. Thus it would not be very unusual to observe 30% surviving in 10 patients (corresponding to the null hypothesis) even for an active regimen. As such, we would probably not want to decide we had sufficient evidence to conclude the new regimen inactive with only 10 patients. Furthermore, while it is important to be able to stop a trial early when the regimen is inactive, it is also important to be conservative early, in order to guard against rejecting an active agent due to treating a chance series of poor risk patients. In order to balance this concern with the concern of treating the fewest possible patients with an inactive agent, at the first stage we test H_1 at the 0.02 level. This is conservative (we mistakenly reject active agents early at most 2% of the time), while at the same time making it possible to stop early when nothing is happening.

A second consideration in our choice of a standard design was that it can take a long time to complete a trial with multiple stages. Typically after the first stage of accrual we do not have enough information to determine whether the criterion for continuing to the second stage has been met, and the study has to be temporarily stopped in order to get this information. After closure, it can take several months for sufficient follow-up to determine the endpoint for each patient, more time for data to be submitted and records to be reviewed, and yet more time to process the reopening. For reasons of practicality, this consideration motivates the use of no more than 2 stages of accrual.

Third, although some alternative designs specify early stopping of a Phase II trial for positive results, we have found that circumstances for which this option is important are rare. In addition, if early results appear positive, there is no ethical concern about accruing additional patients. This increased accrual allows further documentation of the level of activity, as well as a more precise understanding of the profile of adverse events. Moreover, a subsequent protocol for further testing of an agent found to be active is rarely in place at the end of a phase II trial. Thus our standard Phase II trial design stops trials early only if the alternative hypothesis is rejected (for inactivity); we do not stop early if the null is rejected (for activity).

A fourth justification for our standard design is that the percent of new agents found to be active is not high in cancer, which suggests that designs should have fairly high power and fairly low significance level (see discussion in the section on randomized vs single-arm designs below).

An appealing property of the SWOG standard design is that decision guidelines correspond reasonably well to intuition as to what constitutes evidence in favor of one or the other of the hypotheses. Stopping at the first stage occurs when the estimate of the response probability is less than approximately p_0, the true value that would mean the agent would not be of interest. At the second stage the agent is concluded to warrant further study if the estimate of the response probability is greater than approximately $(p_0 + p_1)/2$, which typically would be near the historical probability expected from other agents, and represents the value at which one might be expected to be indifferent to the outcome of the trial.

A final point to make concerning our standard design is that multi-institution studies cannot be closed after precisely a specified number of patients has been accrued. It takes time to get a closure notice out, and during this time more patients will have been approached to enter the trial. Patients who have been asked and have agreed to participate in a trial should be allowed to do so, and this means there is a period of time during which institutions can continue registering patients even though the study is closing. Furthermore, some patients may be found to be ineligible after the study is closed. We try to time study closures carefully, but it is rare we get the precise number of patients called for by the design. We need designs that are flexible enough to be used when the exact sample size isn't attained. One of the advantages of the SWOG standard designs is that they are easily applied when the attained sample size is not the planned size. What we do is apply a 0.02 level test of the alternative at the first stage to the attained sample. If this is rejected, the trial is not continued; if it is accepted, the trial is continued to the second stage. After the second stage, the final test of the null hypothesis is done at the design specified level using all patients accrued. This approach has been investigated analytically and shown to have reasonable properties compared to other possible approaches to the problem (Green and Dahlberg, 1992). In the SWOG S0415 example, sufficient numbers survived longer than 6 months in the first stage, so accrual was continued to the second stage. The final sample size was 55 eligible patients, with 20 patients surviving 6 months, below the 23 in the protocol specified cut-off, so the regimen was concluded to have insufficient activity in this patient population.

5.1.2 Other Single-Arm Phase II Designs

Various other two-stage (or more) Phase II designs have been proposed (Simon, 1987; Fleming, 1982; Chang et al., 1987; Simon, 1989; Simon and Wittes, 1985; Liu et al., 1993). Some (e.g., Simon, 1989) minimize the expected number of patients required on study subject to specific restraints. A problem with these designs is that sample size has to be accrued exactly, so in practice they can't be carried out in most settings. Adaptive modifications of the designs in Fleming (1982) and Simon (1987) are possible (Green and Dahlberg, 1992). The framework for these Phase II designs involves selection of specific null and alternative hypotheses that are useful for determining sample size, and defining rules for declaring whether or not an agent or regimen is of interest for further testing. Ultimately, estimates of the outcomes of interest (percents or medians) and confidence intervals are the most important study outcomes (see Chapter 8).

5.1.3 Alternative Endpoints

Although the most common applications of Phase II trials in the past relied on the traditional measure of response (a categorical outcome) as the study endpoint, adaptations are possible for different endpoints. As noted in the S0415 example above, OS (and PFS) endpoints can be categorized by comparing, for example, 6-month PFS or OS between the experimental arm to the same statistic from a historical population. Alternatively, there are modifications of these methods that allow comparison of median PFS or OS (see Tangen and Crowley, 2006). In all cases, the key issue is whether there is an appropriate choice of a historical control value. Where this is not well known, alternate designs should be considered.

5.1.4 Single-Arm Pilot Designs

Single-stage designs (or "pilot studies") may be acceptable if the regimen being studied consists of agents already shown to be active. In this case, the ethical concern about treating patients with ineffective treatment doesn't apply. Goals for pilot studies are often feasibility (e.g., "Can this regimen be given in a cooperative group setting with acceptable toxicity?") or estimation (e.g., "What is 2-year survival to within $+/-10\%$?"), in addition to the usual goal of deciding whether or not to continue testing the regimen. Sample sizes for pilot studies are typically 50–100 patients, depending on how precise the estimates need to be.

5.2 Multi-Arm Phase II Trials

5.2.1 Nonrandomized Phase II Designs with a Control

Sometimes studies are done using a control group selected from similar patients treated in the past. A study (NHL-BMF95) of the utility of prophylactic cranial radiation therapy (PCRT) in children and adolescents with lymphoblastic lymphoma provides an example (Burkhardt et al., 2006). Stage III-IV CNS-negative patients with sufficient day 33 response from two previous trials from the same investigational group (NHL-BMF 86 and 90, on which patients received PCRT) were selected for comparison to 156 patients with the same characteristics on the new trial who did not receive PCRT (only 6 patients received PCRT on the new trial). Treatments on the three trials were quite similar, although induction chemotherapy differed to an extent (daunorubicin dosing was changed as was the L-asparaginase dose and manufacturer). Patient characteristics were also similar, although there was more mediastinal disease and a lower percent of patients with precursor B cells on the previous studies. For the new trial 86% of patients were event free at 2 years versus 91% in the control patients. The 95% lower confidence bound for the difference was −11%, which met the prespecified criterion to conclude PCRT might not be necessary given the serious late risks of the procedure. Cumulative incidences of CNS failure were similar in the groups, although non-CNS failure was somewhat lower in the BMF90 part of the control group. In the discussion the authors note the importance of interpreting results critically due to use of an historical control group. Various issues are outlined, including an acknowledgment that some bias might have been introduced due to use of a lower L-asparaginase induction dose on BMF95. The authors are also careful in their conclusion: "For CNS-negative patients with stage III or IV LBL and sufficient response to induction therapy treatment without PCRT may be noninferior to treatment including PCRT." This is in refreshing contrast to so many small trials assessed against a previous sequence of patients with a conclusion of "no difference" when results are nonsignificant. See, for example, Cheung et al. (2008) who conclude "adding daclizumab to a tacrolimus-based therapy is safe but cannot further improve clinical efficacy," based on 36 patients who received experimental treatment compared to a previous sequence of 21 patients who did not; this despite an observed higher rate of primary endpoint failures (acute rejection of cadaveric renal transplants) in the control group.

Since results of the control group are already known, design considerations are different when a retrospectively controlled trial group is included instead of a prospective one. In this case, sample size considerations are a function of the known results. Designs may also account for covariate adjustment to help control potential bias (Makuch and Simon, 1980; Dixon and Simon, 1988; O'Malley et al., 2002; Lee and Tseng, 2001).

5.2.2 Randomized Phase II Designs with a Control

A single-arm Phase II trial is only as good as the reliability of the historical information and the suitability of the choice for the null hypothesis. As trials have moved away from response endpoints, as standard treatments have changed, and as knowledge of tumor types have identified more selected subsets for study, the confidence in the selection of a null hypothesis based on historical controls has diminished. This has resulted in an increased emphasis on the conduct of randomized Phase II trials with randomization between the new regimen and a control arm. In many cases, these trials no longer involve new INDs as single agents, but as additions to control regimens.

TABLE 5.1

Comparison of Sample Size Requirements for Single-Arm and Randomized Phase II Trials

Control Median (in months)	Experimental Median (in months)	Type I Error/Power for Randomized Phase II	Sample Size for Randomized Phase II	Type I Error/Power for Single Arm Phase II	Sample Size for Single Arm Phase II
6	9	0.10/0.80	126	0.05/0.90	60
		0.15/0.80	99	0.10/0.90	42
12	18	0.10/0.80	131	0.05/0.90	62
		0.15/0.80	102	0.10/0.90	48
18	27	0.10/0.80	154	0.05/0.90	73
		0.15/0.80	120	0.10/0.90	56

To accommodate the multi-arm nature of these kinds of trials, some compromises have to be made in order to maintain a relatively small sample size for these Phase II trials. Thus, the Type I and II errors can no longer be held to 5% and 10% (as in the standard SWOG single-arm designs) and must be made much larger. Rubinstein et al. (2005) present some proposals for choices of sample sizes and error rates that might be appropriate for a study with either a binary endpoint, or a time to event endpoint, where levels of 15%–20% and power of 80% are proposed to help maintain relatively small sample sizes (they use the term "screening design" for their proposal). As an example, SWOG S0727, a randomized Phase II trial in metastatic pancreatic cancer, evaluated the targeted agent IMC-A12, a monoclonal antibody directed at the insulin-like growth factor receptor family (IGF-1R). The trial compared PFS in patients treated with the standard of gemcitabine and erlotinib to patients treated with these two agents combined with IMC-A12. The study design called for accrual of 106 patients, sufficient to detect a hazard ratio of 1.5 (corresponding to a change in PFS from 2 months to 3.5 months) tested at one-sided 10% Type I error, and 90% power. (Note that these same parameters could have been tested in single-arm design using 54 patients if the historical control data were felt to be accurate). Table 5.1 gives sample sizes for various choices of outcome for randomized versus single-arm designs under various scenarios, for a time-to-event outcome.

5.2.3 Randomized Selection Designs

In some cases the aim of a Phase II study is not to decide whether a particular regimen should be studied further, but to decide which of several new regimens should be taken to the next phase of testing (assuming they can't all be). In these cases "selection designs" may be used. Patients are randomized to the treatments under consideration, but the intent of the study is NOT a definitive comparison. The intent is to choose for further study a treatment which you are pretty sure is not worse (or at least not much worse) than the other new treatments. The decision rule from a selection design is often formulated as "Take on to further testing the treatment arm observed to be best (by any amount)." The number of patients per arm is chosen to be large enough that if one treatment is superior by γ, and the rest are equivalent, the probability of choosing the superior treatment is π. This formulation means if one of the treatments is substantially superior, it will probably be chosen for further testing. If there isn't one that is substantially superior, the chosen one may not be the best, but it will probably be within at most γ of the best. It must be stressed that this design does not result in the conclusion that the selected treatment is better than the others, only that it is the best bet for further testing.

Sample sizes for selection designs have been worked out both for response endpoints (Simon et al., 1985) and survival endpoints (Liu et al., 1993). For example, if there are two treatment arms and one wants a 90% chance (π) of selecting the better arm with respect to response when the probability of response is 0.15 (γ) higher on one arm than the other, at most 37 patients per arm are required. If there are three arms, at most 55 per arm are required; if four arms, 67. For survival as an endpoint, γ is expressed in terms of hazard ratios (see Chapter 2 for a discussion of hazard functions and hazard ratios). The required sample sizes for a 90% chance of selecting the best arm when $\gamma = 1.5$ are 36, 54, and 64, respectively for two, three, and four arms (under the assumptions of exponential survival, maximum follow-up time approximately twice the median survival of the inferior arms, and equal amounts of time for accrual and additional follow-up).

One important characteristic of selection designs is that an arm is always chosen. The potential for difficulty is clear. If one of the regimens is superior, but by less than γ, the procedure may miss it and choose another. If more than one regimen is very promising, the procedure will choose only one. If all of the regimens are poor, the procedure still picks one. If at the conclusion of a study no regimens are chosen because they all looked too poor, then the assumptions on which the statistical considerations were based would no longer hold. The probability that an arm superior by γ would have been chosen would now be less than π (since an option not to choose a regimen superior by γ was added after the fact). Ignoring the design in one respect leaves open the possibility that for other outcomes it would have been ignored for other reasons. It would be impossible to figure out what might have been concluded under other circumstances, and therefore impossible to figure out what the probability of choosing a superior arm really was. If the properties of a trial are unknown, it is very difficult to interpret the trial—thus these designs should probably not be used unless one is quite committed to continued testing of the best arm in a subsequent study.

A modification to the selection design to require that the "winning arm" above must satisfy some minimum success (compared to some historic information) in order to be taken on for further testing is given in Liu et al. (2006). This was used in SWOG S0342, which tested two sequencing strategies in advanced non-small cell lung cancer (Herbst et al., 2010).

5.2.4 Other Randomized Designs

One design popular among researchers is what is sometimes also called a "screening design," but otherwise termed "parallel noncomparative regimens." This is often confused with the "selection" design described above. However, in this design, patients are randomized between multiple experimental arms, but not directly compared to each other. This can essentially be viewed as running parallel single-arm Phase II trials, each to be compared to a historical control value (Mandrekar and Sargent, 2010). Alternatively, a control arm could be added to the design, with parallel comparisons of the control arm to each treatment arm. Design pros and cons are similar to those of the single-arm or randomized-control arm designs discussed in Section 5.4, with the additional need to inflate the sample size to accommodate the multiple testing.

SWOG trial S8905, with its seven variations on 5-FU in advanced colon cancer, is an example of a screening trial that didn't work well. This may have been an appropriate setting for a selection approach as described above; unfortunately, the goals were more ambitious, testing was more complicated, and results were largely inconclusive. The seven arms were (1) 5-FU IV push (standard treatment), (2) low-dose leucovorin plus 5-FU IV push, (3) high-dose leucovorin plus 5-FU IV push, (4) 28 day continuous infusion 5-FU, (5) leucovorin plus 28 day continuous infusion 5-FU, (6) 5-FU 24 hour infusion, and (7) PALA plus 5-FU 24 hour infusion. The design (described as a Phase II-III screening design) called for 80 patients per arm, with comparisons of each of the six variations versus standard 5-FU, plus comparisons of arms 4 versus 5 and 6 versus 7. Each test was to be done at the two-sided 0.05 level, with power 0.67 for each to detect a 50% improvement in survival due to one of the arms. Any of arms 4–7 with no responses after the first 20 patients accrued was to be dropped (Phase II part). There was sufficient experience with arms 2 and 3 that a Phase II aspect was not required for these. After the Phase II testing was complete, four interim analyses and a final analysis were planned for each two-way comparison remaining (Phase III part). It was anticipated that a large confirmatory trial would follow using the regimens showing encouraging survival trends. Various difficulties with the design are evident. In spite of being labeled as a Phase II/III trial, this study was not designed with appropriate power to justify a Phase III conclusion. The overall level is a problem with so many pairwise 0.05 level tests. If only one of the eight primary comparisons in this trial were significant, it would be difficult to claim that the result was particularly encouraging. The overall power is a problem as well. Suppose there were 50% improvements for 1 versus 2, 4 versus 5, and 6 versus 7. Since these comparisons involve different patients, results are independent (see Chapter 2) and the power to detect all three differences is calculated by multiplying $0.67 \times 0.67 \times 0.67$, resulting in a power of only 0.3. Another problem is that the design did not specify how early stopping or the final conclusion would be handled if the two-way tests, taken together, were inconclusive (e.g., 7 significantly better than 1, but not significantly better than 6, and 6 not significantly better than 1). The trial results were inconclusive. No encouraging trends were observed (let alone statistically significant differences). Only arm 7 could fairly clearly be ruled out as ineffective (Leichman et al., 1995). A follow-up Phase III trial comparing arms 4 and 6 was negative, and without a standard 5-FU control arm, no conclusion regarding improvement over standard therapy was possible.

Another version of randomized Phase II designs is termed the randomized discontinuation design. In this type of study, patients are all treated during a "run-in" phase to the experimental arm. Only those patients in whom disease remains stable at a designated time point (and who have not experienced serious adverse events) are then randomized between the experimental arm and either a placebo or standard treatment. The argument for this type of design is that the randomized group will be more homogeneous, having eliminated those with rapidly progressing disease, and thus that the randomized portion of the study may require fewer patients. Unfortunately, these designs are also hard to interpret if the true objective is to estimate treatment effects. Both "arms" require patients to have succeeded during the run-in. Thus, any estimate of effect is based on this condition. There is no information on the differential treatment effect if all patients had first been given the standard arm, or if a lack of difference in the randomized arms is due to the fact that a true effect of the new treatment only manifests itself early, with little yield from longer term treatment. Further, the sample size may need to be substantial in order to accrue enough randomized patients.

5.3 Other Phase II Designs

5.3.1 Multiple Endpoint Designs

There are also designs for Phase II studies that formally incorporate both response and toxicity into the decision rules (Bryant and Day, 1995; Conaway and Petroni, 1995). For these designs both the number of patients with tumor response and the number with acceptable toxicity must be sufficiently high to conclude the regimen should be tested further. Although these are perceived as a good compromise, they rely not only on specification of null and alternative hypotheses for each individual outcome, but for some "joint" relationship between them as well. Moreover, when toxicity is one of the endpoints, identifying a single measure of toxicities can be difficult. Thus, the establishment of decision rules in these designs between two qualitatively different outcomes seems arbitrary. We think it best to base the design on a primary endpoint, then use judgment about how secondary endpoint information should be used to evaluate the agent or regimen is tested further.

Other designs address multiple endpoints using a three-outcome approach instead of the usual two (response or no response). Zee et al. (1999) propose assessing both response and early progression, requiring both a high proportion of responses and low proportion of early progressions. Other variations on this theme include proposals to address CR, PR, and no response (Panageas et al., 2002) or response, prolonged stable, and failure (Lin et al., 2008). An application of the multinomial approach of recent interest is that of window designs. These involve treatment of newly diagnosed patients with a new regimen for a short period prior to the start of standard therapy. The assumption is that use of patients not compromised by prior treatment may improve the chance of identifying active regimens. However, a concern is that delay of standard treatment may put patients at risk. Thus a multinomial outcome of response, no response, and early failure is typical (Chang et al., 2007). Due to the risk, settings in which such trials are suitable should be considered carefully; also consider that short-term use of the agent (typically 4–12 weeks) might not be sufficient for assessing efficacy.

5.3.2 Multi-Strata Trials

An alternative to doing separate trials of an agent or regimen in various subsets (for example, several histologic types of sarcomas) is to do a single trial including all the subsets, with an analysis plan that includes borrowing information across subsets, rather than regarding them as independent. The potential advantage is a saving in sample size with little loss in power, provided there is in fact a relation between the subsets in terms of outcome. Thall et al. (2003) present an approach using Bayesian hierarchical modeling, while LeBlanc et al. (2009) give a frequentist design featuring separate stopping rules for the overall and within subset results. A more complicated design with subsets defined by marker groupings, and multiple treatments, is the BATTLE trial (Kim et al., 2011).

Another approach to stratified design is proposed in London and Chang (2005), and Sposto and Gaynon (2009). Null probabilities of response for each stratum are specified and the number of responses observed in the trial are tested conditional on the number of patients accrued in each stratum. A challenge for this approach is estimating the proportion of patients who will be accrued to each stratum. If the estimates are off, the sample size may also be off and power may be higher or lower than expected. Note that conclusions regarding each stratum cannot be made with this design, but for a trial with a heterogeneous population this is potentially a more useful approach than postulating a single null probability.

5.4 Randomized versus Single Arm: The Pros and Cons

Randomized Phase II designs are not new. What has changed is the increased emphasis on these designs. What has made them so pervasive? A clue to the push toward randomized Phase II trials comes from recent experience in studies of pancreatic cancer. This disease, with a median survival of 6 months for patients diagnosed with advanced/metastatic disease, has seen few advances in treatment. The current standard treatments are based on a gemcitabine backbone, but even the original data supporting this agent were based on a small clinical trial that used a definition of clinical benefit to justify the outcome (Burris et al., 1997). During the first decade of the 21st century, three separate Phase III trials were completed by different cooperative groups. Each of these trials was developed based on "promising" results from single-arm Phase II trials (Xiong et al., 2004; Kindler et al., 2005; Louvet et al., 2002) and each compared gemcitabine to gemcitabine plus the new agent of choice: cetuximab (Philip et al., 2010), bevacizumab (Kindler et al., 2010), and oxaliplatin (Louvet et al., 2005 and Poplin et al., 2009). In each case the subsequent Phase III trials failed to show improvement on the experimental arms. This lead to the conclusion that there was a problem with using single-arm Phase II trials to guide the Phase III designs. However, these results may not be so surprising. Zia et al. (2005) reported on 43 Phase III trials following Phase IIs in the same population with the same treatment. In 35 of the 43 trials, response rates were lower than in the Phase II trial; in only one was the response rate substantially higher than the Phase II result. Worse, even under these best of circumstances with the Phase II trial being done in the same population with the same treatment, only 12 of the 43 Phase III trials were positive. It is likely that treatments not taken to Phase III would have fared even worse, but this is not an encouraging rate of success.

Was the fault with the Phase II trials in these examples? Or is the problem that few agents are really useful, meaning that many positive Phase II results are false positives?

Simon (1987) summarized response results for 83 NCI sponsored investigational agents. In the solid tumor Phase II studies the observed response probability was greater than 0.15 in only 10% of the 253 disease/drug combinations tested. Thus, at the time of this older study approximately 10% of new cytotoxic regimens were estimated to be truly active. We do not have similar estimates for targeted agents, but it is reasonable to assume this number to be approximately the same. In this situation, how do the choices of level and power influence the chance of taking forward to Phase III an agent that is really not active? Table 5.2 gives the probability of identifying true positives under varying scenarios. Thus, for example, with level 15% and 80% power, less than 40% of the agents identified as positive and taken to Phase III would be true positives. Changes in level have much more influence than changes in power. Note that this table is independent of sample size (and independent of whether the study is a single-arm or randomized Phase II), and relates only to the choice of error rates, and assumptions about the overall number of true positive agents being tested. Thus, if the population being studied has a reasonable choice for a historical control, it is feasible to select a sample size for a single-arm trial that can have tighter choices of level and power, limiting the number of false positive trials that move forward. This fact is little appreciated in the push for randomized Phase II trials for all situations.

One of the premises of randomized Phase II trials is that one gets an unbiased estimate of the effect size of the new treatment. But this is at the cost of

TABLE 5.2

True Positive Probability in Phase III Following
Positive Phase II

Type I Error	Power	Probability of True Positive
0.15	0.8	37%
	0.9	40%
0.10	0.8	47%
	0.9	50%
0.05	0.8	64%
	0.9	67%

much higher sample sizes. A simulation study by Taylor et al. (2006) evaluated this issue, and determined that when there is little or modest bias in the choice of historical values, the single-arm trial is more efficient than doing a randomized trial. More recently Tang et al. (2009) showed how patient drift over time can adversely impact the use of single-arm trials. Thus, a key issue in a design decision is the reliability of the historical data. Where the bias is not of great concern, the trade-off becomes one of practicality. Randomized Phase II trials require 2–4 times the sample size, with often high compromises in level and power. Does this guarantee more accurate predictions of successful Phase III follow-up trials?

As described above, Zia et al. reported a low Phase III success rate after positive Phase II trials that should have been predictive (same population, same treatment). Factors that might contribute to low success rates include inappropriate choice of the null hypothesis for the Phase II, insufficiently precise estimates of response or other outcomes due to small sample sizes, and insufficiently conservative testing resulting in too many false positive results. Other factors include change from academic institutions to community settings with potential for more poor risk patients, and use of a short term primary endpoint that may not be very predictive of the Phase III endpoint. Simply randomizing does not address most of these factors, but does address the problem of inappropriate choice of the null hypothesis.

If an accurate value for the null hypothesis is available, then a single-arm trial is the best choice for a Phase II study. Consider a single-arm trial of 50 patients testing 0.25 versus 0.45 with level approximately 0.05 and power 0.9. For a randomized Phase II trial to have similar level and power as the single-arm trial, 200 patients are required. Of course 0.25 will not be correct in every study. Assume for example that 0.25 is correct for 40% of trials, that it is 0.35 in 40% of trials and 0.15 in the remaining 20% of trials, due to variations in the types of patients accrued. In this case the single-arm approach results in 21% false positive results instead of 5% and the power is reduced to 86%. For the 200 patient randomized trial, the level stays at 5% and the power is 88%. Let us further assume that 20% of new treatments are active with respect to response, that half of these produce a survival benefit, and that in addition a small percent of agents inactive with respect to response will still have a survival benefit. Then in 100 trials using the single-arm Phase II approach, 34 Phase IIIs (one-sided 0.025 level with power 0.9) will be done and 9 will be positive. Using the 200 patient randomized Phase II approach, 22 Phase IIIs will be done and 9 will be positive. The large randomized Phase II approach yields a higher success rate in Phase III, but this is at the expense of doing Phase IIs that may be large enough to be termed Phase III. Single-arm trials yield the same number of positive Phase IIIs. More Phase IIIs are done than for the large randomized Phase II strategy, but the single-arm Phase IIs require $\frac{1}{4}$ of the patients and are completed more quickly. Thus even with moderate uncertainty in the historical probability, the single-arm strategy may be a reasonable option.

In settings where there is limited historical information a large randomized Phase II may be justified, both for better decision making and because improved estimates for control patients will be important for the design of future studies. Otherwise it is not so clear that use of randomized Phase IIs will improve decision making. Consider carefully how reliable historical estimates are and what sort of approach to limiting errors might be best for the particular disease and treatment under study.

Clearly the single-arm Phase II runs into problems where there is little control information, where there have been rapid changes in the standard of care, or there are drifts in the types of patients being studied. This is especially true for rare tumor types, or where a study is designed for a new patient subset, perhaps based on treatments for patients selected for targeted therapy based on the presence of a marker, or high levels of expression of a marker. In these cases, randomized Phase II designs may be the most appropriate. However, there may still be value in a single-arm trial to assess feasibility, or to look for a very large signal in a small population, with the goal of assessing further in a larger Phase II setting. This strategy might increase the percent of agents that are truly positive for evaluation in randomized Phase II trials. Some general guidelines for use of randomization in Phase II trials are given in Rubinstein et al. (2009).

5.5 Conclusion

In this section we have discussed some of the issues we consider in deciding on a Phase II design. A final note on Phase II designs is a reminder that the selected primary endpoint is just one consideration in the decision to pursue a new agent. Other endpoints (such as survival and toxicity, if response is the primary endpoint) must also be considered. For instance, a trial with a sufficient number of responses to be considered active may still not be of interest if too many patients experience life threatening toxicity, or if they all die quickly; or an agent with an insufficient number of responses but a good toxicity profile and promising survival might still be considered for future trials.

6

Phase III Trials

On the 20th of May 1747, I took twelve patients in the scurvy, on board the Salisbury at sea. Their cases were as similar as I could have them. They all in general had putrid gums, the spots and lassitude, with weakness of their knees. They lay together in one place, being a proper apartment for the sick in the fore-hold; and had one diet common to all ... Two of these were ordered each a quart of cyder a-day. Two others took two spoon-fuls of vinegar three times a-day ... Two others took twenty-five gutts of elixir vitriol three times a-day, upon an empty stomach; using a gargle strongly acidulated with it for their mouths. Two of the worst patients ... were put under a course of sea-water ... Two others had each two oranges and one lemon given them every day. These they ate with greediness, at different times, upon an empty stomach ... The two remaining patients, took the bigness of nutmeg three times a-day, of an electuary recommended by an hospital surgeon ...

The consequence was, that the most sudden and visible good effects were perceived from the use of the oranges and lemons; one of those who had taken them, being at the end of six days fit for duty.

—James Lind (1753)

Leaping ahead a couple of millennia from Daniel, we find "the first deliberately planned controlled experiment ever undertaken on human subjects" (Stuart and Guthrie, 1953), a six-arm trial with two patients per arm. The study is a tremendous improvement over the biblical "trial." It was painstakingly planned, including efforts to eliminate bias (except that two of the worst got seawater), and was reported in sufficient detail to judge the quality. Despite the pitifully small sample size, the correct conclusion, that citrus prevented scurvy, was reached. Lind was fortunate that one of his treatments produced a cure. We, having to live with modest treatment effects and high variability, need to consider the problems in conducting comparative trials.

6.1 Randomization

As noted in Chapter 3, randomization ensures that patients are assigned to treatment arms without systematic differences in baseline characteristics. The goal is to have good balance between treatment arms for important characteristics thought to affect outcome. When the sample size is large, simple randomization achieves this balance on average for both known and unknown characteristics. Because there is no guarantee this will occur, and because at interim analysis even a large randomized trial can be small, most trials use randomization schemes which help control the balance for selected factors.

6.1.1 Stratification Factors

Stratification factors should be those known to be strongly associated with outcome. If the number of participating institutions is small, it may be best to stratify on this factor as well, since standards of care may differ by institution. However, any randomization scheme will fail to produce balance if there are too many factors included. In general, we suggest no more than three stratification factors given the sample sizes generally used in cancer clinical trials.

   If it is considered possible that the size or direction of treatment effect will be substantially different in two subsets of patients, then stratification is not sufficient. Subset analyses with sufficient sample size in each subset (in effect, two separate studies) will need to be planned from the beginning.

   Various schemes are used and have been proposed to achieve both random treatment assignment and balance across important prognostic factors. The randomized block design is perhaps the most common. In this scheme, the number of patients per arm is equalized after every block of patients; within the blocks the assignment is random. Stratification is achieved using this scheme by having blocks within specific types of patients. For instance, if a study is to be stratified on age (<40 vs. 40–60 vs. 60+) and performance status (0–1 vs. 2), then blocked randomization would be done within each of the six defined patient groups.

   Note that the number of groups increases quickly as the number of factors increases. Four factors with three categories each result in 81 distinct patient groups, for example. In a moderate-size trial with multiple factors, it is likely that some groups will consist of only a few patients—not enough to complete a block—so imbalance can result.

   Dynamic allocation schemes often are used to solve this problem. Instead of trying to balance treatment within small patient subsets, the treatment assigned (with high probability) is the one that achieves the best balance overall across the individual factors. Balance can be defined in many ways. A common approach is due to Pocock and Simon (1975). For example, consider a study with two factors (sex and race) and two treatment arms (1 and 2) and several patients already entered. The factors for the next patient registered are male and white. The Pocock-Simon approach involves computing, for each of the two possible treatment assignments, the number of white patients and the number of males that would result on each arm. The patient is assigned

TABLE 6.1

Control of Imbalance as a Function of Number of Factors

Measure of imbalance, $N = 400$.			
Factors	Simple Randomization	Randomized Blocks	Dynamic Allocation
2	13.8	1	0.8
8	13.8	7.8	1.4
12	13.8	13.5	1.6

with high probability (e.g., 2/3) to the arm that would achieve the smaller overall imbalance.

Table 6.1 shows how well simple randomization, randomized blocks and dynamic allocation schemes do in a two-arm, 400 patient trial with increasing numbers of factors (Therneau, 1993). The numbers in the table are a measure of the variability in imbalance—the smaller the number, the closer to balance a trial is likely to be. Simple randomization does not force balance, so variability remains high for any number of factors. Randomized block schemes do well with small numbers of factors but become similar to simple randomization as the numbers increase. Dynamic allocation schemes also increase in variability with the number of factors but much more slowly.

Apart from balance of the selected factors, stratification has other benefits. For instance, balance on unknown factors cannot be worse than with simple randomization (Aickin, 2001) and may be better, for example for factors correlated with the stratification factors. Furthermore, balancing reduces the variability of the estimate of the difference between treatment arms, so results in more efficient studies. Weir and Lees (2003) did simulations based on a cardiac trial and estimated an 8% increase in effective sample size by using a stratified approach instead of simple randomization. Begg and Kalish (1984) had similar results from simulations based on five ECOG studies; results suggested reduced efficiency of simple randomization compared to stratified allocation with estimates of relative efficiency from 92% to 99%. (Note that there is no efficiency gain if the factors chosen are not, in fact, associated with the endpoint.)

Each randomization scheme differs in emphasis on what is to be balanced. A randomized block design with a small number per block and no factors will result in very nearly equal numbers of patients on each arm, but does not control for chance imbalance in important prognostic factors. A block design within each type of patient defined by the factors achieves the best balance within subtypes of patients, but the number of patients per arm can be badly imbalanced. Dynamic schemes fall in between, but these do not guarantee balance within each subtype of patient (the number of males might be the same on each arm, as well as the number over 40, but males over 40 aren't necessarily balanced).

6.1.2 Timing of Randomization

In general, the best time to randomize is the closest possible time to the start of the treatments to be compared. If randomization and the time of the start of treatment are separated, patients may die, deteriorate, develop complications from other treatments, change their minds, or become unsuitable for treatment, resulting in a number of patients not treated as required. If these patients are removed from the analysis then the patient groups may no longer be comparable, since such deviations may be more frequent on one arm than the other or reasons for deviations may be different on the arms. If all patients eligible at the time of randomization are used in the primary analysis of the study as we recommend (the "intent to treat principle" discussed in Chapter 8), then such complications add unnecessary variability. Thus it is best to minimize the problem by randomizing close to the start of treatment. For instance, in a study of adjuvant treatment for colon cancer, randomization should occur within one working day of the start of chemotherapy rather than at the time of surgery.

Similar considerations apply when the treatment for the two arms is common for a certain period and then diverges. For example, if there is a common induction treatment followed by high-dose therapy for one group and standard therapy for another, randomization after induction therapy eliminates the problems caused when many of the patients don't receive the high-dose therapy. If randomization is at the start of induction, these patients are either improperly eliminated from the analysis, causing bias, or add variability to the real treatment comparison, necessitating larger sample sizes. Randomization before such treatment divergences may be required for practical reasons (e.g., to make obtaining consent easier or to add time for insurance coverage to be guaranteed). Differences in treatment arms may also begin later than the actual start of treatment on a study by choice. For instance, SWOG S7827 compared 1 year versus 2 years of adjuvant chemotherapy (CMFVP) in women with receptor negative, node positive breast cancer (Rivkin et al., 1993). Randomization could have been done at the start of treatment or after 1 year in patients still on CMFVP. Note that the two approaches ask different questions. The first asks if 2 years or 1 year of treatment should be planned from the onset of adjuvant chemotherapy. The second asks if patients who have made it through one year of chemotherapy should be asked to continue for another year. To see the difference, consider Table 6.2, adapted from Rivkin et al.

The decision was made on this trial to randomize at the start of treatment. Even though the first year was supposed to be identical for the two arms, there were some interesting differences observed in the drop-out patterns. Among patients with good-risk disease (one to three nodes involved) more on the 2-year arm dropped out in the first 6 months than on the 1-year arm, while this was not true for patients with poor risk disease (four or more nodes involved). It is possible that knowledge of assignment to 2 years of toxic treatment was a factor in the more frequent decision of good-risk patients to drop out of treatment early, while those at higher risk of recurrence may

TABLE 6.2

Compliance Data by Treatment and Number of Positive Nodes for SWOG 7827

	1–3 Positive Nodes 1-Year Arm	1–3 Positive Nodes 2-Year Arm	4+ Positive Nodes 1-Year Arm	4+ Positive Nodes 2-Year Arm
No. at Risk at 12 Months*	86	92	83	92
Treated < 6 Months	6%	20%	10%	7%
Treated > 11 Months	86%	72%	83%	85%
No. at Risk at 24 Months		78		71
Treated > 23 Months		32%		42%

*No. at risk is the number of patients alive and disease free at 12 months (i.e., those who should have been treated for a year).

have been more motivated (or encouraged more) to continue despite the long haul ahead. One of the conclusions from this study was that two years of treatment was difficult to complete. (In fact it was the main conclusion, since compliance was too poor for the trial adequately to address the benefit of adding a year of treatment.) If the study had been designed to register and randomize patients after 1 year of treatment had been completed, we can speculate that the study would have been closed early due to poor accrual, but no conclusions concerning the difficulty of completion of a planned 2-year treatment course could have been made and no exploration of early drop-outs by randomized arm could have been done.

Another issue in the timing of randomization is when to obtain patient consent. Most often patients are asked to participate before randomization has occurred; part of the consent process is to agree to a random assignment of treatment. In studies of competent adults, this is the only timing we believe is appropriate. It has been argued that "randomized consent" designs are appropriate in some circumstances (Zelen, 1979). In these designs randomization occurs before patient consent, after which the patient is asked to participate according to the assigned arm. (In another proposed version of the design only patients randomized to the experimental arm are asked for consent, while those assigned to the control arm are given control treatment without consent—the reasoning being that control treatment is all that should be expected ordinarily.) A common motivation in considering use of this design is the perception that it is easier to accrue patients to a trial if the assignment has already been made. This leads to the concern, however, that patients do not give a truly informed consent, but rather are subtly persuaded that the arm to which they are assigned is their best choice (Ellenberg, 1984). Apart from the ethical issue, there is also an analytic drawback to this design. It is often conveniently forgotten that patients are supposed to be analyzed according to the assigned arm, not to the arm received or not to be left out of the analysis. If very many patients refuse their assigned treatment, interpretation of the study is compromised.

6.2 Other Design Considerations

6.2.1 One-Sided or Two-Sided Tests

A typical objective in a Phase III trial is "to compare A and B with respect to survival in the treatment of patients with . . . ." As discussed in Chapter 2, the null hypothesis is usually equality of survival distributions (or equivalently, of hazard functions), and the alternative is that survival is not the same. Whether or when the alternative hypothesis should be specified as one-sided or two-sided is a matter of some debate. (This issue is of practical importance, since a two-sided test of the same level requires a larger sample size than a one-sided test in order to achieve the same power.) Some statisticians argue that the alternative should always be two-sided because it is always possible that either arm could be worse. We view the issue more as a decision problem. If at the end of the trial of A versus B the conclusion is going to be either "continue to use A" or "use B," this is a one-sided setting; if the conclusion is going to be either "use A," "use B," or "use either," then it's two-sided. For instance, adding an experimental agent to a standard regimen is nearly always a one-sided setting. At the end of the trial the decision is made whether to use the extra agent or not. If the agent has either no effect or a detrimental effect on survival, the agent won't be used; if survival is improved the agent generally will be recommended for use. It would not be sensible to conclude "use either arm." Furthermore, even though the agent could be detrimental, going out of one's way to *prove* it is harmful is probably unethical. On the other hand, a comparison of two standard treatments is often a two-sided setting. The decision to be made is whether one of the standards should be recommended over the other, or if either is acceptable.

6.2.2 Significance Level, Power, and Sample Size

Choice of significance level (α), power ($1-\beta$), and the difference to be detected are the major determinants of sample size (see Chapter 2). The difference specified to be detected should generally not be what has been observed in other studies, but rather the smallest difference it would be important to detect. A toxic treatment when the standard is no treatment might require a fairly large benefit to be worthwhile, for example. After effective treatments have been identified, however, smaller benefits may be worth detecting.

Concerning choice of significance level, the standard 0.05 is usually reasonable. Occasionally it is important to be more conservative, such as for highly controversial or highly toxic treatments. In these cases it might be prudent to have stronger evidence of effectiveness, perhaps at the 0.01 level instead of 0.05, before recommending the treatment for use.

We consider 80% power to be a bit low, as this means 20% of effective treatments will not be detected. (Specifically, this is 20% of the treatments effective at the specified difference. More than 20% of treatments effective at a level less than that specified will be missed.) Considering that relatively few new treatments are found to be even modestly effective in cancer, we generally recommend 90% power.

When survival is the primary endpoint of a study, differences between arms are usually expressed as a hazard ratio, $R(t)$. The hazard ratio is the ratio of the death rates among those still alive on the two arms at each point in time (see Chapter 2). If the ratio is the same at all times, $R(t)$ is a constant R; this is called the proportional hazards assumption. Exponential survival distributions for all arms of a study give one example yielding constant hazard ratios. (As noted in Chapter 2, a hazard ratio in the exponential case is the inverse of the ratio of median survivals between the arms.) A constant hazard ratio of unity means the death rates at each point in time (and therefore the survival distributions on the two arms) are the same. If survival is very different and the proportional hazards assumption holds, R is either close to zero or very large. The most common hypotheses in phase III trials are formulated statistically as $H_0 : R = 1$ versus $H_1 : R > 1$ or versus $H_1 : R \neq 1$. Rather than give formulas (the formulas are not simple) for sample size when survival is the endpoint, we will give some general ideas on how various factors change the sample size requirements. Besides α, β, and R, the major influence on sample size is the amount of follow-up patients have relative to how long they live. The main point to be made is that the sample size is driven by the number of deaths expected rather than the number of patients accrued. A relatively small study of patients with rapidly lethal disease may have the same power as a very large study of patients with a low death rate and short follow-up. The number of deaths increases as median survival decreases, and as the length of time each patient is followed increases.

Table 6.3 illustrates the effect of level, power, hazard ratio to be detected, median survival, and follow-up on sample size. Assumptions used in the calculations included exponential survival distributions (see Chapter 2) and accrual of 200 patients per year. The formula is described by Bernstein and Lagakos (1978).

TABLE 6.3

Sample Size per Arm Required for a One-Sided Two-Arm Trial under Various Assumptions when the Accrual Rate is 200/Year

		α	$1-\beta$	T	α	$1-\beta$	T	α	$1-\beta$	T	α	$1-\beta$	T	α	$1-\beta$	T	α	$1-\beta$	T
m	R	0.05	0.8	1	0.05	0.8	5	0.05	0.9	1	0.05	0.9	5	0.01	0.9	1	0.01	0.9	5
1	1.25		330			260			430			360			610			530	
	1.5		130			80			170			110			240			170	
	2.0		60			30			80			40			110			60	
5	1.25		640			430			790			570			1050			800	
	1.5		310			160			390			220			510			310	
	2.0		170			70			210			100			280			140	

Note: α is the level, $1-\beta$ the power, R the hazard ratio for which the specified power applies, m is the median survival time in years on the control arm, and T is the number of years of additional follow-up after accrual is complete.

A comparison of the sample sizes presented here compared to those based on the binomial in Table 2.9 is instructive. Researchers often mistake the notion that a change in the survival probabilities at a particular point in time is the same as a change in the hazard ratio. Consider a study for which a "25% increase in survival" is the stated goal. If a 25% increase in the 1 year from survival from 40% to 65% is desired, then according to Table 2.9, 74 patients per arm would be sufficient. However, this change corresponds to a hazard ratio of 2.13, implying that median survival time more than doubles. If instead a 25% increase in median survival is desired (hazard ratio of 1.25) the sample size required per arm is several hundred.

The assumption of exponential survival distributions is common in determining sample size. Real survival distributions are never precisely exponentially distributed, but using the assumption for calculating sample size is generally adequate, provided the proportional hazards assumption still holds, at least approximately (Schoenfeld, 1983). If the proportional hazards assumption is not correct, the standard sample size calculations are not correct (Benedetti et al., 1982). For example, if survival is identical until time t before diverging (hazard ratio 1 followed by hazard ratio $\neq 1$), the standard formulas don't hold. Deaths during the time the curves are identical don't provide information on the difference between the arms, so in this setting sample size is driven by the number of deaths after time t rather than the total number of deaths. Any type of clear divergence from standard assumptions will require a different type of sample size calculation.

6.2.3 Multiple Endpoints

The above discussion addresses studies with one primary endpoint only. Generally we find that the clinical endpoint of greatest importance is easily identified; this then is primary and the one on which the sample size is based. The remaining endpoints are secondary and reported separately. Others have proposed an approach of combining all endpoints using weighted sums of differences of each endpoint of interest (O'Brien, 1984; Tang et al., 1989; Cook and Farewell, 1994). A problem with this approach is that the weights assigned are fairly arbitrary. The investigators make a judgment as to the relative importance of each endpoint (survival, time to progression, toxicity, various aspect of quality of life etc.) and weight the differences observed on the treatment arms accordingly. Since no one puts precisely the same importance on all endpoints, we do not find this approach satisfactory. Instead we recommend reporting each endpoint comparison separately. If the direction of the differences do not all favor the same arm, judgments concerning which is the preferred treatment can be made according to individual preferences.

If claims of significance for secondary endpoints are intended (e.g., for regulatory purposes), then testing strategies that allow for tests of multiple endpoints without compromising the primary comparison should be considered. For instance, a simple gatekeeper approach whereby secondary endpoints are not tested unless the primary comparison is significant could be used. For this and more complex strategies see Dmitrienko et al. (2009). Whatever strategy is used must be specified in the protocol as part of the design; post hoc plans will likely be viewed as inflating level and may compromise interpretation of the trial.

6.3 Equivalence or Noninferiority Trials

Suppose you are reading the results of a randomized clinical trial for which the primary aim was to compare two treatment arms with respect to the probability of response. The study had been designed to detect a difference of 0.15 in response probabilities. At the time of publication, the response on arm A was 25%, only 5% higher than on arm B. The results of the trial were disappointing to the investigators, so they stopped the trial early and concluded there were "no significant differences" between the arms. Does the finding of no statistically significant differences in this study establish clinical equivalence?

The answer most likely is no. *Failure to reject* the null hypothesis is not equivalent to *proving* the null hypothesis. A p-value of 0.9 doesn't mean we are 90% sure the null hypothesis is correct. Recall from Chapter 2 that a p-value P means that the probability of the observed result (or one more extreme) under the null hypothesis is equal to P. A small p-value means the observed result doesn't happen often when the true response rates are identical; a large one means it does happen often. If it doesn't happen often, the evidence contradicts the null hypothesis and we can conclude the treatments are (likely to be) different. If it does happen often, the evidence does not contradict the null hypothesis—but, unfortunately, we cannot in this case conclude the treatments are equivalent. This is because there are other hypotheses that the evidence does not contradict.

To illustrate, consider the initial example, in which the observed percent responding for arm A was 20% and arm B was 25% (a 5% observed difference). Under the null hypothesis $H_0 : p_A = p_B$ (response probabilities on arm A and arm B are equal), the p-value for this observed difference depends on the sample size. Table 6.4 gives the p-values and 95% confidence intervals for a range of sample sizes. (See Chapter 2 for a discussion of confidence intervals.) The largest p-value in Table 6.4 is 0.71, when the sample size is 20 per arm. Despite the large p-value, it is clear from the confidence interval, which covers both -0.15 and 0.15, that the evidence is consistent with a broad range of true values, and that either arm could still be substantially superior. On the other hand, the smallest p-value under the hypothesis of equality occurs at 640 per arm. With this sample size the 5% difference is statistically significant—but this sample size also provides the strongest evidence that the two response probabilities are similar (the confidence interval indicates arm A is better by less than 0.1).

TABLE 6.4

Observed Percents Responding are 25% on Arm A and 20% on Arm B

N per Arm	p-Value for $H_0 : p_A = p_B$	Confidence Interval for $p_A - p_B$
20	0.71	$(-0.21, 0.31)$
40	0.59	$(-0.13, 0.23)$
80	0.45	$(-0.08, 0.18)$
160	0.28	$(-0.04, 0.14)$
320	0.13	$(-0.01, 0.11)$
640	0.03	$(0.00, 0.10)$

Note: Table gives two-sided p-value for testing the hypothesis of equality and the 95% confidence interval for the difference in response probabilities (normal approximation).

Considering the question from another perspective, Table 6.5 shows the observed difference that would be required for the p-value to be approximately the same for each sample size, and the corresponding 95% confidence interval. At 20 patients per arm a p-value of 0.7 means the difference could be as large as 0.3; at 640 patients per arm, the same p-value means the difference is no larger than 0.06. The table illustrates the fact that large p-values for tests of equality provide more evidence for the null hypothesis when sample sizes are large.

It is clear from the tables that the p-value for testing equality does not in itself provide useful information concerning the equivalence of two treatments. How could the authors legitimately claim results are approximately equivalent? One way is by using a different p-value to test a different hypothesis. The authors were interested in detecting a difference of 0.15. That can be tested by making the null hypothesis "the response probability on arm A is superior by 0.15 or the response probability on arm B is superior by 0.15" ($H_0 : p_A \geq p_B + 0.15$ or $p_A \leq p_B - 0.15$). If this hypothesis is rejected, then we can conclude that the response probabilities on the two treatment arms are

TABLE 6.5

Observed Percent Responding is 25% on Arm A

N per Arm	% Responding, Arm B	Difference, Arm B − Arm A	p-Value for $H_0 : p_A = p_B$	Confidence Interval for $p_A - p_B$
20	20	0.05	0.71	$(-0.21, 0.31)$
40	22.5	0.025	0.79	$(-0.16, 0.21)$
80	22.5	0.025	0.71	$(-0.11, 0.16)$
160	23.1	0.019	0.70	$(-0.07, 0.11)$
320	23.8	0.012	0.71	$(-0.05, 0.08)$
640	24.1	0.009	0.70	$(-0.04, 0.06)$

Note: Table gives the % responding on Arm B required to result in a p-value of approximately 0.7 and the 95% confidence interval for the difference in response probabilities (normal approximation).

TABLE 6.6

Two-Sided p-Values for Tests of H_1

N/Arm	$H_1 : p_A = p_B + 0.05$	$H_2 : p_A = p_B + 0.15$	$H_3 : p_A = p_B - 0.15$	CI for $p_A - p_B$
20	1.0	0.45	0.13	$(-0.21, 0.31)$
40	1.0	0.28	0.03	$(-0.13, 0.23)$
80	1.0	0.13	0.002	$(-0.08, 0.18)$
100	1.0	0.09	0.001	$(-0.07, 0.17)$
160	1.0	0.03	0.000	$(-0.04, 0.14)$
320	1.0	0.002	0.000	$(-0.01, 0.11)$
640	1.0	0.000	0.000	$(0.00, 0.10)$

Note: $p_A = p_B + 0.05$, $H_2 : p_A = p_B + 0.15$, and $H_3 : p_A = p_B - 0.15$ for various sample sizes when the observed percent responding on Arm A is 25% and the observed percent on Arm B is 20%

within 0.15 of each other. Table 6.5 shows p-values for testing three different hypotheses, $H_1 : p_A = p_B + 0.05$ (arm A superior by 0.05), $H_2 : p_A = p_B + 0.15$ (arm A superior by 0.15), and $H_3 : p_A = p_B - 0.15$ (arm B superior by 0.15). The 95% confidence interval for the difference in probabilities is also repeated. For $N = 20$, the tests show that the outcome would not be unusual when either arm, in truth, had a response probability of 0.15 greater than the other arm. The test of the hypothesis that arm A is superior by 0.15 is not rejected, and the test of the hypothesis that arm B is superior by 0.15 is not rejected. It is not until 160 patients per arm that the hypotheses are both rejected; this is reflected in the confidence interval which excludes both -0.15 and 0.15. Table 6.6 also illustrates the fact that if you test the observed result, you always get a p-value of 1.0, which should also help convince you that large p-values don't mean much by themselves.

6.3.1 Designing an Equivalence or Noninferiority Trial

The same reasoning that allows us to conclude approximate equivalence when a completed trial is sufficiently large and results are sufficiently close also allows us to design a trial with an equivalence objective (Blackwelder, 1982; Harrington et al., 1982; Kopecky and Green, 2006). Instead of using the standard null hypothesis of no difference, the null hypothesis is phrased instead as a small difference between the arms. The one-side version of equivalence, noninferiority, has become more common as the number of disease settings for which there are useful agents has increased. Alternative treatment options are still desirable in these settings, and if other aspects are favorable, demonstration of superior efficacy of a new agent should not necessarily be required to conclude it is useful. For example, it might be hypothesized that Treatment A is less toxic and has similar efficacy to standard Treatment B. In this case the null hypothesis would be that A is less efficacious than B by an amount Δ (a small loss in efficacy would be acceptable given improved toxicity), and the alternative would be A = B.

The choice of Δ, which is termed the noninferiority margin, has been a topic of considerable discussion. It may be chosen on clinical grounds based on judgment as to acceptable loss of efficacy, or it may be based on the estimated difference, d, between B and placebo. For the latter, Δ cannot be greater than d (otherwise rejection does not preclude A being no better than placebo). It may also not be considered sufficient to choose Δ = d, since in this case rejection of Δ would only suggest A is better than placebo, not necessarily that it is similar to B. Thus margins are chosen to show that at least a fraction of the benefit of B is preserved (FDA Guidance for Industry, 2010); often Δ = $d/2$. If this hypothesis is rejected, the conclusion is not that the arms are the same but that the difference between them is smaller than Δ. A point to note is that the sample size required to rule out a small difference in a noninferiority trial is about the same as that required to detect a small difference in a superiority trial. Consequently, a well-designed equivalence trial will typically be very large.

6.4 Designs for Targeted Agents

Recent decades have seen the development of numerous agents aimed at targeting cellular pathways or other aspects of tumors and their micro-environment that are much more specific to tumors than traditional cytotoxic agents. Examples include trastuzumab, targeted at tumor cells expressing the growth factor Her-2 (particularly for breast cancer patients); erlotinib, targeted at the epidermal growth factor pathway (especially for non-small cell lung cancer); imatinib, developed to attack cells with the bcr-abl translocation that characterizes chronic myelogenous leukemia (but which also is effective for c-kit positive tumors such as GI stromal tumors); and cetuximab, particularly effective for colon cancer patients whose tumors are k-RAS wild type (not mutant).

Testing such targeted therapies presents new challenges for the design of clinical trials. Thus far, we have discussed Phase II and III trials which are designed to test an overall treatment effect for patients of a specific disease type. In theory, then, testing a targeted agent should be no different, with the exception that eligibility now restricts patients to a specific subtype based on expressing the hypothesized target. Unfortunately, the challenge is multifold. For one, sometimes the subpopulation represents a small proportion of the patients, making feasibility a big concern. Moreover, because we typically have little historical experience with outcomes in these subgroups of patients, we necessarily need to design our trials with larger numbers (e.g., randomized as opposed to single-arm Phase II trials) for even early pilot studies. Of greatest concern, many of the purported targets can not be measured accurately, or even at all, and the drug may not hit the target, at least as measured. Thus, the designs of many of the trials that have thus far been conducted are not suitable to the conclusions put forth.

Many pilot studies of markers are conducted in single-arm trials. Based on an observation that a genotype, or a gene expression level (often categorized as high/low) is correlated with outcome in a group of patients treated with an agent of interest, many of the studies concluded that the marker "predicted" which patients benefitted from therapy. Without knowing the relative clinical outcome for patients with this marker profile treated with another agent (presumably not related to the target), there is no way to know whether the marker is just correlated with outcome, and thus a marker of prognosis only, or whether there is indeed a treatment specific link, making the marker predictive of relative treatment benefit. This corresponds to the difference between assessing a main effect for treatment, or for investigating a marker by treatment interaction. As the sample size needed to assess marker by treatment interactions is often quite high, the evaluation of the real predictive benefit of a marker/treatment combination can be quite daunting.

There have been a number of proposals for the design of Phase III trials for targeted agents. Briefly, these designs fall into three general categories: (1) All comers (randomize all) designs. In these designs, all patients have their markers evaluated, but all patients are randomized to the same two (or more) treatments. If it is practical to evaluate the marker prior to randomization, then patients can be stratified by marker value; (2) marker+ (enrichment) designs. In these designs, the marker is evaluated, and only those patients with a prespecified genotype or expression level are eligible for the trial; and (3) strategy designs, where patients are randomized to marker based therapy versus non-marker based therapy.

A successful example of an all comers design is the study done by the National Institute of Canada Clinical Trials Group (Shepherd et al., 2005). Patients progressing after initial chemotherapy for non-small cell lung cancer were randomized to either placebo or erlotinib. The erlotinib arm had a superior survival outcome, leading to regulatory approval of erlotinib for this indication. A retrospective analysis showed that patients whose tumors expressed high levels of the target for erlotinib, the epidermal growth factor receptor (as measured by immunohistochemistry), had marked benefit, while those whose tumors were negative had no apparent benefit. Not all patients had tissue readily available for analysis (one reason the all comer and not the marker+ design was used); these patients as a group had intermediate benefit from erlotinib.

The trial of trastuzumab in patients with advanced breast cancer, which lead to regulatory approval of this agent, used the marker+ design (Slamon et al., 2001). The marker, Her-2, as measured by immunohistochemistry, is positive in only about 20% of patients, making the marker+ approach the only practical one (see explanation below).

The most basic version of the strategy design randomizes patients between a "standard treatment," and one based on targeted assignment, in which patients with positive marker values are assigned to the proposed targeted therapy and the remainder to the standard. The analysis compares all patients on the "strategy" arm to all those on the standard arm. For many, the allure of this approach is the idea that they are testing "strategy" versus not. Unfortunately, the question is more complicated. First, this design means that a portion of the patients on the strategy arm (marker negative patients) are being treated with the same agent as those on the standard arm. As a result, any potential improvement in outcome for those getting the targeted therapy will be diluted. In addition, this design assumes that the targeted agent only works for patients with the hypothesized "correct" marker profile. If the agent could also be useful for all patients, this will not be detected (this is also a drawback of the marker+ design). A final drawback to these designs occurs if marker results are only obtained for those patients assigned to the targeted assignment arm. In this situation, patients who do not have available specimens, or in whom the specimens cannot be evaluated may be allowed on the standard arm, but not the strategy arm. Knowledge of the marker status on the standard arm would allow at least a comparison directly between treatments for the targeted patient subset.

One of the first studies of this type was conducted by Cobo et al. (2007), a Phase III trial using expression levels of the excision repair cross-complementing 1 (ERCC-1) gene to assess the preferential use of gemcitabine over cisplatin in patients with non-small cell lung cancer. The targeted arm assigned patients with low ERCC-1 levels to docetaxel/cisplatin, while those with high ERCC-1 received docetaxel/gemcitabine. The control group all received the docetaxel/cisplatin regimen. Although this study can be lauded for its forward thinking (it was conducted in the early 2000s, well before such marker-based studies were being put forth), it suffers from many defects. First, more than 10% of patients randomized to the strategy arm were ineligible due to lack of analyzable tissue. No such restriction was placed on the control arm patients. Second, the primary endpoint was response, and while a comparison of arms showed a statistically significant difference, this result could either be due to the predictive value of ERCC-1, or to intrinsic differences in the treatment regimen. Without knowledge of the ERCC-1 values in the control, and without knowledge of the use of the gemcitabine in the low ERCC-1 cohort, these questions cannot be answered. Moreover, there were no significant differences in overall or progression-free survival.

Various authors have evaluated the pros and cons of these different designs. Simon and Maitournam (2004) evaluated the relative efficiency of marker+ (enrichment) designs compared with the all comers (randomize all) design. They concluded that the marker+ design is most efficient when the underlying biology is well understood, and there is clear reason to limit the study to the subpopulation of interest, and when the marker prevalence is low. However, the assumptions may not hold, and since a large number of patients must be screened in order to find those eligible for the study, this type of design may be less desirable than it first appears. Sargent et al. (2005) studied the all comers and strategy designs and proposed variations on the strategy design meant to be used for combined regulatory approval of a marker assay (device) and the associated targeted therapy.

Hoering et al. (2008) investigated the power of the three basic designs under a number of different scenarios, including cases where the cutpoint for marker positivity is not well established. Marker negative patients might have some benefit, or might even be harmed, by the targeted therapy. They concluded that where the marker cutpoint value is known and the treatment only effects the true positives, then the marker+ is the most powerful. Where the new treatment might help marker negative patients, or where the cutpoint has not been well established, or where marker prevalence is high, the all comers design is preferred. They show the strategy design is inefficient in all cases considered.

SWOG study S0819 in advanced non-small cell lung cancer uses an important variation on the all comers design. Patients are randomized to standard chemotherapy + cetuximab, which targets the epidermal growth factor receptor. Measurement of the target is done by fluorescence in situ hybridization. One comparison is between the two randomized groups (all comers), but in addition there is a comparison between patients who are marker positive in the two groups. Each comparison is done with a smaller Type I error so that the overall study false positive rate is preserved.

As part of the analyses leading to the final design for S0819, sample sizes for various alternatives were calculated, for fixed assumptions of power 0.90 for a 20% overall improvement in progression free survival, with one-sided Type I error 0.025 (Redman, 2012). Marker prevalence was assumed to be 40%. The sample size required for the all comers design is 1340 patients, while the marker+ design requires 1380 patients to randomize 522 (this assumes a 33% improvement in the marker positive subset). The strategy design takes 2888 patients. However, if the all comers comparison is done with Type I error 0.02 instead of 0.025, and the comparison for the marker positive subset is done at level 0.008, the overall false positive rate of 0.025 is preserved, there are two chances for a positive outcome (overall and in the subset), and the number of patients is only increased to 1430 patients, from 1380.

Targeted designs rely on technology to produce reliable and reproducible assays. A review by the Colon Cancer Working Group of the Program for the Assessment of Clinical Cancer Tests (Taube et al., 2005) reviewed more than 100 articles of what at the time were the most promising results identifying possible markers for predicting outcome in colon cancer. Most of these studies were determined to be too small, used inconsistent assays, and yielded conflicting results. This, coupled with a general lack of validation studies, dampened enthusiasm for any recommendations to bring these markers forward in clinical trials. Thus, an important question is not just which kind of design to use, but perhaps more importantly, when is a marker ready for evaluation at all?

6.5 Multi-Arm Trials

The frequent use of the standard two arm randomized clinical trial is due in part to its relative simplicity of design and interpretation. At its most basic, one power, one level, and one magnitude of difference to be detected have to be specified to determine sample size. Conclusions are straightforward: either the two arms are shown to be different or they are not. When more than two arms are included, complexity ensues. With four arms, there are six possible pairwise comparisons, 19 ways of pooling and comparing two groups, and 24 ways of ordering the arms (not to mention the global test of equality of all four arms), for a grand total of 50 possible hypothesis tests. Some subset of these must be identified as of interest; each has power, significance level, and magnitude considerations; the problems of multiple testing have to be addressed; and drawing conclusions can be problematic, particularly if the comparisons specified to be of interest turn out to be the wrong ones.

6.5.1 Types of Multi-Arm Trials

The simplest extension of the two-arm trial is to a comparison of K treatments, where no systematic relationships among the treatments exist and all comparisons are of interest. For instance, SWOG study S8203 (Cowan et al., 1991) compared three similar drugs—doxorubicin, mitoxantrone, bisantrene—in advanced breast cancer. None of the arms was hypothesized to be superior, and all three pairwise comparisons were of potential interest in this study.

Sometimes trials are designed with specified relationships hypothesized among the arms. Common examples in this category would be studies designed with order restrictions among the treatment arms, such as arms with increasing doses, or arms with successively added agents. SWOG lung study S8738 (Gandara et al., 1993) is an example of a multi-arm study with ordering— patients were randomized to receive standard-dose CDDP, high dose CDDP, or high dose CDDP plus mitomycin-C, with survival hypothesized to improve with each addition to therapy.

In studies of a control versus multiple experimental arms, one of the treatments to be compared is a standard arm or control arm while the remaining arms are promising new treatments. The intent is to determine if any of the new treatments are superior to the control arm. For example, SWOG lymphoma study S8516 compared standard CHOP chemotherapy to three regimens that had shown promise in nonrandomized trials (MACOP-B, mBA-COD, and ProMACE-CytaBOM—all more toxic and more expensive than CHOP) in stage II non-Hodgkin's lymphoma, in order to determine if the new generation regimens were superior to CHOP, and, if so, which new regimen was best (Fisher et al., 1993). "Screening" designs are related to control versus multiple experimental designs, but occur earlier in the development of the experimental regimens (see Section 5.2.4).

One special type of multi-arm trial is the factorial design, in which two or more treatments (possibly at multiple dose levels) are of interest alone or in combination. A factorial design assigns patients to each possible combination of levels of each treatment. Often the aim is to study effect of levels of each treatment separately by pooling across all other treatments. SWOG study S8300 in limited non-small cell lung cancer provides an example for a factorial design (Miller et al., 1998). In this study, the roles of both chemotherapy and prophylactic radiation to the brain were of interest. All patients received radiation to the chest and were randomized to receive prophylactic brain irradiation (PBI) plus chemotherapy versus PBI versus chemotherapy versus no additional treatment. PBI was to be tested by combining across the chemotherapy arms (i.e., all patients with PBI—with or without chemotherapy—were to be compared to all patients without PBI), and chemotherapy was to be tested by combining across PBI arms.

Designs with multiple randomizations are related to factorial designs, but one or more interventions occur at later times among those still on study, or among selected subsets of patients. For instance, SWOG study S8600 (Weick et al., 1996) initially randomized patients with acute myelocytic leukemia to standard-dose chemotherapy versus high-dose chemotherapy; then among standard-dose patients in complete response the study randomized again to standard-dose versus high-dose.

To illustrate the issues in designing multi-arm trials, the above SWOG examples will be used, along with a simulation study (Green, 2006) that investigated a four-arm trial of an observation only group O versus Treatment A versus Treatment B versus A and B (AB). The simulated trial had 125 patients per arm accrued over 3 years and 3 additional years of follow-up. Survival was exponentially distributed on each arm and median survival was 1.5 years on the control arm. The sample size was sufficient for a 0.05 level test of A versus not-A to have power 0.9 for a hazard ratio of 1.33 when there was no effect of B.

6.5.2 Significance Level

Multi-arm trials give rise to problems due to the inherent desire to test multiple hypotheses. Each test done in a multi-arm trial has an associated significance level (probability of rejecting the null hypothesis when it is true). If each test is performed at level α, then there will be a probability greater than α that at least one comparison will be significant when the null hypothesis is true, resulting in an experiment-wise significance level greater than α. If many tests are done, the probability can be much greater than α. For instance, when all 50 tests mentioned in the introduction were done on 1000 simulated four-arm trials with no differences among the arms, there were "significant" results (at least one test significant at the 0.05 level) not in 5% of the trials, but in 28%. (In 10% of the trials 11 or more tests were "significant"!)

A common approach to this problem is to start with a global test (test of equality of all arms), followed by pairwise tests only if the global test is significant. Doing a global test before allowing yourself subset tests helps limit the probability of false positive results. An alternative method is to adjust the level at which each test is performed. For example, if K tests are planned, each test could be done at level α/K. This so-called Bonferroni correction results in an experiment-wise level of no more than α.

In other multi-arm settings it is not necessary to adjust for all possible tests. A limited number of tests may be designated before the trial starts as being of primary interest. All other tests are considered exploratory— i.e., used to generate hypotheses to be tested in future studies, not to draw firm conclusions. Statisticians disagree on the issue of whether the primary questions should each be tested at level α, or whether the experiment-wise level across all primary questions should be α. Regardless of one's statistical philosophy, however, it should be kept in mind that if the experiment-wise level (probability of at least one false positive result in the trial) is high, a single positive result from the experiment will be difficult to interpret, and may well be dismissed by others as being inconclusive.

For lung study S8300 investigators chose to design the trial to have level 0.025 for two tests: a test of whether brain RT improved survival and a test of whether chemotherapy improved survival. No other tests were specified. It was assumed that brain RT and chemotherapy would not affect each other. Under these restrictions, the level was at most 0.05 for the experiment.

6.5.3 Power

For power (the probability of rejecting the null hypothesis when a specific alternative is true) in pairwise comparisons, the sample size calculations are the same as for a two-arm trial of the selected arms. However, while specified alternative hypotheses for pairwise comparisons may be reasonable, the pattern of alternatives might be implausible. For instance in a trial of A versus AB versus ABC, the power to detect a difference Δ might be specified for both A versus AB and AB versus ABC, but 2Δ may be an implausible difference between A and ABC. If in truth the differences between A and AB and between AB and ABC are both $\Delta/2$ (for a plausible difference of Δ between A and ABC), then the trial will have inadequate power to detect either the A versus AB difference or the AB versus ABC differences and the results of the trial are likely to be inconclusive.

Power and sample size considerations for ordered alternatives will depend on the method of analysis being proposed. A global test chosen to be sensitive to ordered differences can be used (Liu and Dahlberg, 1995; Liu, Tsai, and Wolf, 1998). The power in this analysis setting often refers to the power of the global test under a specific alternative. A "bubble sort" approach is also a possibility (Chen and Simon, 1994). In this method treatments are ordered by preference, e.g., A > B > C, in the sense that if survival is the same on all three then A is the preferred treatment; B is preferred if B and C have the same survival and are better than A; and C is preferred only if it is superior to both A and B with respect to survival (preference may be due to toxicity or cost, for example).

The testing is done in stages. C versus B is tested first; B is eliminated if the test significantly favors C, otherwise C is eliminated. If C is eliminated, B versus A is tested and B is eliminated if not significantly better than A, otherwise A is eliminated. If B is eliminated after the B versus C comparison instead, C versus A is tested, with C eliminated if not found to be significantly superior to A, A eliminated if it is. The treatment of choice is the one remaining. The power with this approach refers to the probability of identifying the correct treatment arm under specific alternatives. The referenced papers have details on how to determine sample size.

If an aim of the study is to combine certain arms and compare the resulting groups (e.g., combine all arms with agent A and compare to the combination of all arms without agent A), then under certain assumptions it is legitimate to calculate power according to the number of patients in the combined groups. The primary assumptions are (1) other factors and treatments are balanced across the groups (e.g., in both A and not-A there should be the same percent of patients receiving B and the same percent of good and poor risk patients) and (2) the magnitude of the effect of A versus not-A is the same in the presence or absence of all other treatments in the trial (e.g., if there is a 33% improvement due to A in patients not receiving B, there should also be a 33% improvement due to A in patients who are receiving B). In statistical terms this latter condition corresponds to "no interaction" (see next section). Even if both conditions are met, the power for detecting a difference due to A may be decreased if B is effective, due to the decreased number of deaths in patients treated with B. If the usual logrank test (Chapter 2) is used there is additional power loss, which can be substantial. The additional loss is due to the change in shape of survival curves when groups with different distributions are mixed. Logrank tests work best when the proportional hazards assumption is true. Unfortunately, if A versus B differences are proportional and C versus D differences are proportional, it does not follow that the difference between a mixture of A and C versus a mixture of B and D is also proportional—so the logrank test no longer works as well. Use of a stratified logrank test (stratifying on the presence or absence of the other treatments) avoids this additional loss.

The influence on the power to detect an effect of A when B is effective in a trial of O versus A versus B versus AB is illustrated in Table 6.7. The table shows results from the simulation example. If, as is appropriate, a stratified logrank test is used (stratifying on the presence of B for a test of the effect of A), the influence is not large unless B is highly effective. The planned power of 0.9 for a hazard ratio of 1.33 due to A remains above 0.8 even when B is 3 times

TABLE 6.7

Power to Detect a Hazard Ratio of 1.33 due to A

B hazard ratio	1	1.25	1.33	1.5	2	3	4
Power for A, logrank test, unstratified	0.92	0.90	0.89	0.88	0.82	0.76	0.70
Power for A, logrank test, stratified on B	0.92	0.90	0.90	0.89	0.85	0.83	0.81

as effective as A. When an unstratified logrank test is used (inappropriately), the power decline is worse.

Another potential concern is joint power for both A and B. The power to detect a specified effect of A might be 0.9 and the power to detect a specified effect of B might also be 0.9, but the power to detect effects of both A and B can be considerably lower. The simulation again provides an example. If A and B are both effective with hazard ratios 1.33, the probability that both will be identified is only 0.79.

6.5.4 Interaction

The most common analytic strategy used with factorial designs in cancer clinical trials involves collapsing over other factors to test the effect of a given factor. The simplest case is of a 2×2 factorial design, with factor A and factor B, each at two levels, such as in the example above. Collapsing over the presence or absence of B to study A and vice versa seems to be a neat trick—two answers for the price of one—until one considers how to protect against the possibility that the effect of A versus not-A is NOT the same in the presence or absence of B. If the differences between treatments O and A, and B and AB are the same, then combining O with B and comparing to A combined with AB (using a stratified test) is proper. However, it is generally more plausible to assume A will not behave precisely the same way in the presence of B as in the absence of B. This is known as a treatment interaction (and differs from the concept of drug interactions, used to refer to the adverse events caused by the joint administration of certain agents). These interactions can be illustrated by the examples in Tables 6.8 and 6.9, which show two possible scenarios, each with individual treatment effects on median survival for treatments A

TABLE 6.8

Example of Treatment Effects for A and for B, but No Interaction

	B	No B	Hazard Ratio
A	16	12	1.33
No A	12	9	1.33
Hazard ratio	1.33	1.33	Interaction $= 1.33/1.33 = 1.0$

Note: Entries are median survival in months.

TABLE 6.9

Example of Treatment Effects for A and B, and an Interaction

	B	No B	Hazard Ratio
A	21	12	1.75
No A	12	9	1.33
Hazard ratio	1.75	1.33	Interaction $= 1.75/1.33 = 1.32$

and B. In Table 6.8, both of the experimental agents improve median survival. However, the improvement with drug A is of similar magnitude (1.33) whether or not the patient also receives drug B. Similarly, the effect of B is the same whether or not the patient has received agent A. The ratio of either of the two individual hazard ratios is an estimate of the interaction. In this case, $1.33/1.33 = 1$, indicating no treatment interaction. In contrast, in Table 6.9, the effect of Treatment A differs depending on whether or not the patient receives Treatment B. With B, the hazard ratio is 1.75, compared to 1.33 without. Thus, while in this case agent A is useful no matter what, its effect is improved with the addition of B. The corresponding interaction is 1.32.

A useful way to describe interactions is by the following proportional hazards model (see Chapter 2),

$$\lambda(t, x_1, x_2) = \lambda_0(t) \exp(\alpha x_1 + \beta x_2 + \gamma x_1 x_2),$$

where $x_i = 0$ or 1 depending on the absence or presence of A or B, respectively. Figure 6.1 shows the survival distributions for the four arms when A is effective treatment (α is negative), B is not effective (β is 0), and there is no interaction ($\gamma = 0$, where γ is the log of the hazard ratio for interaction). Figures 6.2 and 6.3 illustrate the distributions when A is effective and B is not, but there are interactions. When γ is negative, the AB arm does better than A alone; when it is positive it does worse.

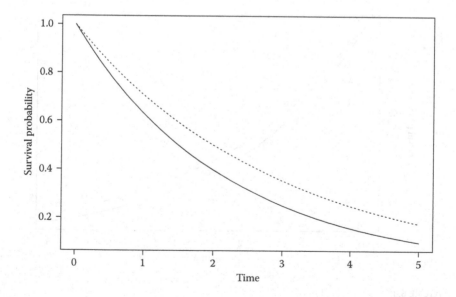

FIGURE 6.1
Survival distributions for a four-arm trial when A is effective, B is ineffective, and there is no interaction. Solid line represents survival distribution for Arms B and control, dotted line represents Arms A and AB.

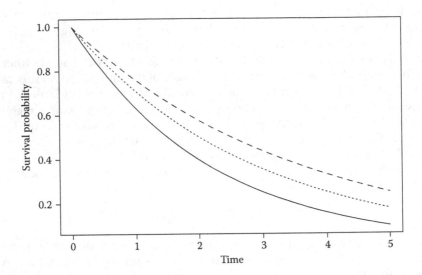

FIGURE 6.2
Survival distributions for a four-arm trial when A is effective, B is ineffective, and there is a
positive interaction. Solid line represents survival distribution for Arms B and control, dotted
line represents Arm A, and dashed line represents Arm AB.

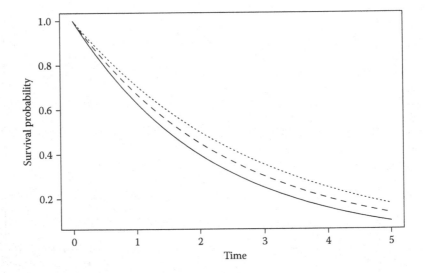

FIGURE 6.3
Survival distributions for a four-arm trial when A is effective, B is ineffective, and there is a
negative interaction. Solid line represents survival distribution for Arms B and control, dotted
line represents Arm A, and dashed line represents Arm AB.

Testing whether there is a significant interaction (testing $\gamma = 0$ in the model) is not often a satisfactory answer. The power to detect interactions is poor, and it is not even clear how to analyze a study when a test for interaction is planned. If there is a plan to test for an interaction, there must also be a plan of how to proceed if the interaction is significant. For instance, if an interaction is significant and indicates that the combination of A and B is not good, then A and B must be tested against O separately. If both are better than O then the question becomes which of A or B is better. Once other analyses are included in the analysis plan, the simple power calculations for testing A versus not-A no longer hold. In fact, the properties of the procedure become complex and difficult to calculate.

Possible approaches to analyzing a factorial design might include (1) pretending interactions don't exist and just testing main effects (A versus not-A and B versus not-B) regardless of results (if both main effects are significant, this leads to a choice of AB), or (2) first doing a global test of the multiple arms and proceeding with other comparisons only if this test is significant, or (3) starting with a test of interaction and proceeding with subset tests if the interaction is significant or main effects if not significant. These approaches were examined in the simulation study from the point of view of identifying the best treatment arm. The choices for "best arm" are: Use O, use A, use B, use AB, or use A or B but not AB. Several observations were made. First, overall significance levels (probability of not choosing O when there is no positive effect of A or B) for approaches 1 and 3 above (just testing main effects, or testing interactions first) are too high (0.11 and 0.13, respectively). Approach 2 (first doing a global test) does restrict the overall level, but this is at the expense of a reduced probability of choosing the correct arm when the four arms are not sufficiently different for the overall test to have high power. Second, when there are no interactions, then testing for one is detrimental. The probability of choosing the correct regimen is reduced if Approach 3 is used instead of Approach 1 when there is no interaction. Third, if there is an interaction you may or may not be better off testing for it. If the interaction masks effectiveness of the best regimen it's better to test for interaction (e.g., when A is effective, B is ineffective and γ is positive; then the best arm is A, but the improvement due to A appears too small when the arms are combined). If the interaction enhances the effectiveness of the best arm, testing is detrimental (e.g., when A is the best arm and γ is negative; then combining arms improves power, but testing for interaction first will mean arms are combined less often). Fourth, the power for detecting interactions is poor. Even using 0.1 level tests, the interactions were detected at most 47% of the time in the simulations. Fifth, all approaches were inadequate for determining the best treatment arm. For each there were plausible clinical scenarios where the probability of choosing the correct arm was less than 0.5 despite the best arm having the desired 33% improvement over the control arm. Finally, interactions that result in decreased effectiveness can wreck a study if any treatments are effective. The probability of identifying the correct regimen is poor for all methods if γ is positive and the correct arm is not the control arm. Approach 1, assuming there is no interaction, is particularly poor. (The probability is 0 in the case where A and B are both effective but the combination isn't, since this approach will lead to choosing A, or to choosing B, or to choosing AB, but not to the choice of "use A or B but not AB.")

Negative interactions and detrimental effects happen: SWOG study S8300 is an unfortunate example. In this study, PBI was found to be detrimental to patient survival. The worst arm was PBI plus chemotherapy, followed by PBI, then no additional treatment, then chemotherapy alone. Using the design criteria (test PBI at the 0.025 level combining across chemotherapy assignment, and test chemotherapy at the 0.025 level combining across PBI assignment), one would conclude that neither PBI nor chemotherapy should be used. With this outcome, however, it was clear that the comparison of no further treatment versus chemotherapy was critical—but the study had seriously inadequate power for this test, and no conclusion could be made concerning chemotherapy.

If power within subsets of treatments is important for any outcome, then a larger sample size is needed. In fact, to protect fully against the possibility of interaction, *more* than twice the sample size is required—four times as many patients are necessary for testing an interaction as for testing a single main effect (A versus not-A) of the same magnitude (Peterson and George, 1993). This clearly eliminates what most view as the primary advantage to factorial designs. A theoretical discussion of factorial designs is presented in a paper by Slud (1994).

6.5.5 Other Model Assumptions

Any model assumption can result in problems when the assumptions are not correct. As with testing for interactions, testing other assumptions can either be beneficial or detrimental, with no way of ascertaining beforehand which is the case. If assumptions are tested, procedures must be specified to follow when the assumptions are shown not to be met, which changes the properties of the experiment and complicates sample size considerations.

The second SWOG lung example (S8738) provides an example where some of the planned analyses were invalidated by other results. The trial was closed approximately halfway through the planned accrual because survival on high-dose CDDP was convincingly shown not to be superior to standard-dose CDDP by the hypothesized 25% (in fact, it appeared to be worse). A beneficial effect of adding Mitomycin-C to high dose CDDP could not be ruled out at the time, but this comparison became meaningless in view of the standard-dose versus high-dose comparison.

6.5.6 Sequential Randomization

Clinical trials with an induction randomization (to get patients into response) and a maintenance randomization (to improve survival after response to induction) are related to factorial designs. If the comparisons of A versus B for induction therapy and C versus D for subsequent maintenance therapy are both of interest, a decision has to be made as to when to randomize to C and D. A trial designed with randomization to C and D done at a later time than the one for A versus B asks a different question from one designed to randomize C and D at the same time as A and B. With respect to C and D, the first asks, "Given patients have completed induction, are still eligible and agree to continue, should C or D be given next," while the second asks, "Which of the planned sequences—A followed by C, A followed by D, B followed by C, or B followed by D—is the best sequence?"

Unless nearly everyone goes on to the maintenance treatment, results using either approach can be difficult to interpret. When randomizations are separated in time, it can be difficult to answer long-term questions about the first randomization. Problems of potential treatment interactions (as for factorial designs but starting later in time) are compounded by patient selection biases related to how different the patients from A and B are who make it to the second randomization. For the same reasons, if A is found to be better than B and C better than D, it can't necessarily be concluded that A followed by C is the optimal sequence. For instance, if D is highly effective after both A and B, and more A patients agree to randomization, then the long-term comparison of A versus B will be biased in favor of A. Or, if A is a better therapy (patients survive longer on A alone than B alone and more patients make it to randomization), but patients induced with B do better on D, the interaction plus the excess of A patients at the second randomization could result in the conclusion that A followed by C is superior, even though B followed by D might be the best sequence.

If both randomizations are done up front, then noncompliance can be a major problem—if patients don't get C or D as assigned, they must still be analyzed according to the assignment. For instance, if there are many refusers and more good risk patients refuse to go through with C while more poor risk patients refuse D, then any differences observed between C and D will be due both to treatment and to the type of patient who chooses to comply with treatment. Although it is still a valid test of the planned sequence, it can be very difficult to interpret. Comparing only those who get the assigned treatment is not valid. Baseline characteristics are balanced only at the time of the initial randomization; if patients are omitted later based on outcome (compliance is an outcome), all benefits of randomization are lost. If the patients who got D were good risk patients and those who got C were poor risk, D is going to look good regardless of effectiveness (see Pater and Crowley, 2006).

The SWOG leukemia committee addressed these difficulties in study S8600 by specifying separate randomizations for induction and consolidation, a short-term endpoint for the induction treatment (complete response) and a long-term endpoint for maintenance (survival). The objectives of the study (comparing high- and low-dose chemotherapy with respect to induction of CR, and testing whether maintenance therapy with high-dose chemotherapy improves survival of patients in CR) can be achieved by the design. Long-term comparisons of induction and sequence questions, although of interest, are not listed as objectives, as they cannot be addressed adequately by the design.

SWOG myeloma study S8229 (Salmon et al., 1990) had objectives difficult to address in a single design. Comparisons with respect to long-term end-points of both induction therapies and maintenance therapies were specified. Both randomizations were done prior to induction therapy. Of approximately 600 patients randomized to induction, only 180 went on to >75% remission and their randomized maintenance assignments, 100 to VMCP and 80 to sequential hemi-body RT plus VP. By the design, VMCP and RT should have been compared using all 600 patients according to their assigned arms, but with 420 patients not receiving the assignments, this would have been uninterpretable. The 100 VMCP patients were compared to the 80 RT patients, but due to all the possible selection biases, this analysis also could not be interpreted adequately.

6.5.7 Concluding Remarks on Multi-Arm Trials

The main points of this section can be summarized as follows:

1. When there are more than two treatment arms, many questions are asked and many tests are done. Multiple tests mean multiple opportunities for errors. Limiting the probability of error when a large number of errors is possible requires a large number of patients.

2. Power calculations depend on model assumptions. More arms require more assumptions. If the assumptions are wrong, the calculations are in error, and the trial may not have adequate power to answer anything of interest. Unfortunately, assumptions are often wrong. Thus, the more arms, the higher the likelihood that the trial will provide no answers.

3. Interactions are common. In fact, it seems plausible that A does NOT work the same way in the presence of B as in the absence of B for most treatments B. When there are interactions, the ability to identify the best treatment arm from a factorial design can be severely compromised. There is a school of thought, led by some statisticians, that advocates the use of factorial designs on the grounds that they deliver something for nothing (two for the price of one in the case of the 2×2 factorial). In our opinion this is tantamount to selling snake oil. Factorial designs were developed in agriculture and have been heavily used in industrial settings when several factors at several levels must be considered with a limited number of experimental units (often no more than 2 per group) in a short amount of time (and never with censoring). In this setting highly structured (factorial or fractional factorial) designs provide the only hope of getting any answers at all. The medical setting could hardly be more different.

4. For the best chance of a straightforward conclusion at the end of a study, use a straightforward design. A series of two-arm trials will

not ask many questions, but will provide answers to most of them (if sample sizes are adequate); a series of multi-arm trials of the same total sample sizes will ask many questions, but can easily result in clear answers to none. If accrual is slower than expected, a two-arm trial might succeed in answering one question while a multi-arm trial may answer none.

5. If there are compelling reasons to consider multi-arm trials, keep in mind the potential problems due to multiple testing, interactions, other incorrect assumptions and noncompliance. Make sure the objectives can be accomplished by the design. Consider what might be salvageable from the study if the assumptions are wrong. Allow room for error by increasing the sample size over that required for the simplest assumptions—this could make the difference between a wasted effort and a surprising result.

6.6 Interim Analyses

Suppose you are conducting a trial of standard fractionation RT versus hyper-fractionated RT in lung cancer and the data are looking interesting halfway through the trial. You decide to do a test and find the logrank test of survival has p-value 0.05. Is it legitimate to stop the trial at this point and conclude that hyperfractionation is superior to standard fractionation?

The answer is no. As explained in Chapter 2, if the difference between two treatment arms is tested at the end of the trial at the 0.05 level, the chance of concluding they are different when, in fact, they are not, is 5%. If this same trial is tested halfway through, by plan, as well as at the end, the chance at the halfway point is also 5%. But if you consider the chance of concluding there is a difference AT EITHER TIME, then the chance is greater than 5%. (If the first analysis is done not by plan but just because the results look interesting, then the overall chance of concluding there is a difference at either time is MUCH greater than 5%.)

Interim analyses are dictated by the ethical imperative that a study be stopped if there are dramatic results in favor of one treatment over another. However, frequent analysis of the data can seriously compromise the trial. Only well-planned interim analyses allow appropriate monitoring while maintaining the integrity of the trial design.

To illustrate the effect of interim analyses, a computer simulation was performed of 100 two-arm trials designed to have a final analysis at year 4 and an interim analysis at year 2. In all 100 trials, the results on the treatment arms were generated from the identical distribution. Five of the simulated studies had differences significant at the 0.05 level at year 4, and five had significant differences at year 2 (Fleming et al., 1984). This is what was expected according to the definition of level 0.05. (And no, there was no cheating. It did indeed come out with exactly the expected number of differences!) The interesting point of this simulation was that none of the studies significant at the 2-year analysis were the same as the studies significant at 4 years. Thus, of the 100 studies, a total of 10 showed significant differences despite no true difference between the treatment arms, yielding an overall Type I error of 10%, not 5%. The 2-year p-values for the studies with apparently significant differences at 2 years were 0.02 in three cases and 0.01 in two; by year 4 these had increased to 0.83, 0.53, 0.13, 0.21, and 0.17. The simulation illustrates both that many early positive results will become negative with further follow-up if there are no true differences, and that the Type I error rate with multiple tests is high. If you test twice, you're going to make a mistake almost 10% of the time instead of 5%; if more testing is done, the chance is even higher, up to as much as 25% when testing is done frequently.

Figure 6.4 shows a real example of a trial inappropriately closed early from SWOG. Figure 6.4a shows how the study looked at the time the apparently inferior arm was dropped. There appeared to be a striking benefit to treatment arm A in the good risk subset of patients. This was based on only a few patients and very short follow-up. Further follow-up saw additional deaths in the good risk arm A patients, and even further follow-up showed that no long-term survivors were in the group. Figure 6.4b shows later results. Differences are no longer of interest. The example illustrates that the patterns of early data can be deceptive.

The statistical solution to the interim testing problem is to use designs that allow for early stopping but that still result in the probability of a false positive conclusion being 0.05 overall. One way to accomplish this is to use designs that limit the number of times the data are tested, and that are very conservative when interim tests are done. Instead of stopping a trial whenever a p-value is 0.05, stop only when p-values are considerably below 0.05 at a few prespecified times (Haybittle, 1971). SWOG standards for stopping trials early are to use 1–3 interim analyses with small and approximately equal probabilities of stopping at each interim time (Crowley et al., 1994). Sample designs are shown in Table 6.10. For instance the first row in the table specifies a design with one planned interim analysis. For this design the study would be stopped early if the difference were significant at the 0.01 level. Otherwise the study would be continued to completion, and the final analysis would be done at the 0.045 level to adjust for the fact that one analysis had already been done. The overall level for this design, and for all of the designs in the table, is approximately 0.05.

In addition, we stop trials early not only when we have highly significant positive results, but also when we have highly significant negative results, done by testing the alternative as a null hypothesis. If there is convincing evidence early on that an experimental regimen is not going to be useful, then the trial should be stopped, particularly if the experimental regimen is more toxic. We don't believe it is necessary to prove a more toxic experimental regimen is actually more lethal than standard treatment before deciding it should not be pursued, only that it is unlikely to have the hoped for benefit. This is the clearest example we know of the virtue of one-sided (asymmetric) testing. A

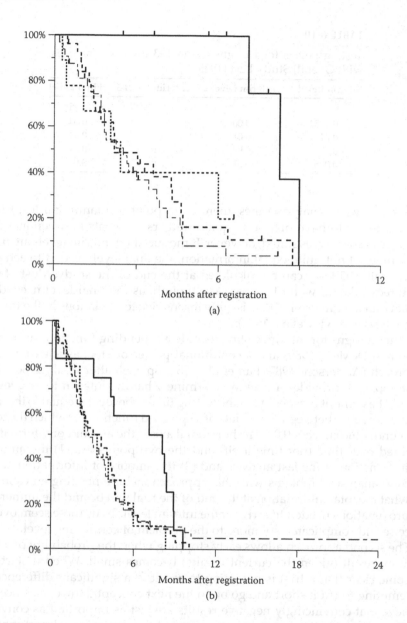

FIGURE 6.4
A trial inappropriately closed early: (a) interim analysis; (b) final analysis. Solid line represents good risk patients on Treatment A.

two-sided approach would stop only if the new treatment were significantly worse; a one-sided approach would lead to earlier stopping based on the new treatment not being better.

Generally interim analyses should be planned after intervals during which a reasonable number of events are expected to occur. (If nothing is going to

TABLE 6.10

Testing Levels for Designs Using 1–3 Interim Analyses,
with Overall Study Level 0.05

Interim Level 1	Interim Level 2	Interim Level 3	Final Level
0.01			0.045
0.005	0.005		0.045
0.01	0.015		0.04
0.005	0.005	0.005	0.045
0.005	0.01	0.01	0.04

happen between analysis times, there is no point in planning a test.) It is
not necessary to have precisely equal numbers of events between analysis
times, as is sometimes stated, however. If the specified interim levels are used
after times of not-quite-equal information, the final level needed to achieve
an overall 0.05 level can be calculated at the end of the study. Most of the
time recalculation won't be necessary, though, as the final level needed to
achieve an overall level of 0.05 is quite insensitive to deviations in the timing
of analysis (Crowley et al., 1994).

Other designs for interim testing include a "spending function" approach
(Lan and DeMets, 1989) and a conditional power or stochastic curtailment
approach (Anderson, 1987; Lan et al., 1982; Spiegelhalter et al., 1986). The
first approach provides a way to determine what the interim testing levels
should be without prespecifying the testing times: the level is equal to the area
under the curve between two points of a specified function for which the total
area under the curve is 0.05. The horizontal axis is the amount of information
accrued over time (not time itself) and the two points are (1) the amount
of information at the last analysis and (2) the amount of information at the
current analysis. Problems with this approach include needing an estimate
of what the total information at the end of the trial will be and the numerous
approximations needed to arrive at the interim level. To us these seem overly
precise and complicated solutions to the problem of controlling level.

The second approach allows early stopping when the probability of a significant result (given the current results) becomes small. When it starts to
become clear that a trial is not going to result in a significant difference, it
is tempting to cut it short and go on to the next concept. However, since we
believe that convincingly negative results are just as important as convincingly positive results, we do not recommend this approach. Unfortunately,
as for large p-values, "is not going to be significant" is also not equivalent to
proving equality.

The concept of "not becoming significant" can be translated statistically as
"conditional power is poor" (i.e., the power to detect a difference given the results so far is poor). Suppose in our example in Tables 6.4 to 6.6 above that the
trial had been stopped after 100 patients per arm had been accrued. Table 6.11
shows the conditional power for various outcomes if the total planned sample
size is 160 per arm, along with the 95% confidence interval for the observed

TABLE 6.11

Conditional Power (Probability of Rejecting the Null Hypothesis of Equality) under the Alternative Hypotheses (1) Arm A Superior with Respect to Response Probability by 0.15 or (2) Arm B Superior with Respect to Response Probability by 0.15 Are True

N per Arm	Arm A Arm B Response %'s	Conditional Power (Arm A by 0.15)	Conditional Power (Arm B by 0.15)	95% Confidence Interval
100 of 160	25, 25	0.08	0.08	(−0.12, 0.12)
100 of 160	25, 22	0.21	0.02	(−0.09, 0.15)
100 of 160	25, 20	0.34	0.01	(−0.07, 0.17)
100 of 160	25, 15	0.73	0.00	(−0.01, 0.21)

Note: Assume 100 per Arm have been accrued out of a total of 160 per Arm planned for the trial.

difference. Despite very poor conditional power when the observed difference is 0.05 or under, the confidence interval only excludes the hypothesized difference of 0.15 when the observed response probability is nearly identical. If the reported difference in response probabilities is > 3%, it is not possible to make a definitive recommendation concerning therapy. The results are consistent either with arm A being better, or with either arm being acceptable. The trial at this point is equivocal, particularly if arm B is less toxic.

Some monitoring strategies include reassessing the required sample size at the time of interim analysis (Gallo et al., 2006). Reassessment may be based on current estimates of various factors such as variability, event rate for the control group, or treatment effect. As for the standard group sequential monitoring plans described above, the key issue for these strategies is to control the Type I error rate. If event rate is uncertain, planning to assess and adjust may be reasonable and error control need not be a problem (Kieser and Friede, 2003). Re-estimations based on currently observed results, however, are problematic for a number of reasons in addition to the error rate issue, such as unreliability of the interim estimate of difference and the potential for too much information to be deducible from the size of the adjustment. Although superficially appealing, these methods are not efficient and standard group sequential schemes are generally to be preferred (Tsiatis and Mehta, 2003).

6.6.1 Examples of Interim Analyses

We conclude this section with several examples of monitoring committees in action. The following studies were conducted under the initial monitoring policy devised by SWOG. These illustrate some of the circumstances under which trials are terminated early and some of the factors monitoring committees consider in their deliberations. The first three trials were closed according to stated stopping guidelines, while the next two had to be closed for unanticipated reasons.

6.6.1.1 Stopping Early for Positive Results

SWOG S8795 (Lamm et al., 1995) was a randomized trial of intravesical Bacillus Calmette-Guerin (BCG) versus mitomycin-C in the treatment of superficial bladder cancer. Recent comparisons of BCG with other intravesical agents (thiotepa, doxorubicin) had demonstrated superiority of BCG. Previous randomized trials had failed to show mitomycin-C was an improvement over thiotepa or doxorubicin, but other (small) trials had failed to show BCG an improvement over mitomycin-C. Since mitomycin-C had the highest complete response rate of chemotherapeutic agents studied in early bladder cancer, a trial of BCG immunotherapy versus mitomycin-C was felt by most members of the genitourinary committee to be justified. The primary endpoint in this study was disease-free survival in the subset of patients with resected T_a or T_1 transitional cell disease with no carcinoma-in-situ. The design called for 663 patients in order to have power 0.9 to detect a 35% improvement due to either arm (i.e., hazard ratio of 1.35 or 1/1.35). Stopping guidelines called for interim analyses after 1/4, 1/2, and 3/4 of the expected information at two-sided levels 0.005, 0.01 and 0.01 levels, with the final analysis to be done at the 0.045 level, using the logrank test.

At the first interim analysis the log-rank p-value was 0.001 (Figure 6.5a) in favor of BCG. Toxicity on BCG was more frequent and severe than on mitomycin-C (28% versus 39% with no toxicity and 31% versus 16% with grade 2–3), but there were no grade 4 toxicities. This is the one study where a consensus on closure was not reached and the final decision had to be made by the Group leadership. Arguments against stopping included (1) recurrence of superficial lesions with no worsening of severity is not life-threatening, so the difference did not prove there would be long-term benefit to the more toxic BCG [a reasonable argument] and (2) no trial would be available to patients if this one closed [not so clearly reasonable—we do hope that patients get superior care on a clinical trial, but this may instead be an example where Group interests and patient interests are not necessarily the same.] Arguments in favor of stopping were (1) a striking difference in the stated primary endpoint was observed and the stopping guideline was met, (2) the study confirmed other evidence that BCG was efficacious in superficial bladder cancer, and (3) the degree of toxicity was not unacceptable. The trial was stopped in favor of BCG. At the time of publication, differences had decreased (Figure 6.5b) as would be expected, but were still significant at $p = 0.02$.

6.6.1.2 Stopping Early for Negative Results

Study S8738 (Gandara et al., 1993) was a trial of high-dose cisplatin, with or without mitomycin-C, versus a control arm of standard-dose cisplatin, in patients with advanced non-small-cell lung cancer. The design called for 200 patients per arm, to achieve power of 0.825 to detect hazard ratios of 1.25. Interim analyses were planned at 1/3 and 2/3 of the expected information, at one-sided 0.005 levels. The final analysis was planned for level 0.045. At

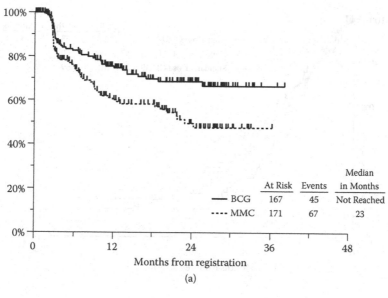

(a)

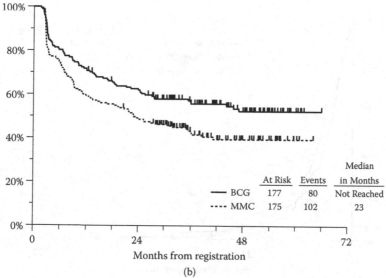

(b)

FIGURE 6.5
Recurrence-free survival in SWOG bladder cancer trial 8795: (a) at time of first interim analysis; (b) at time of publication.

the first interim analysis, roughly halfway through the planned accrual, the alternative hypothesis for the comparison of high-dose to standard-dose cisplatin was rejected with a *p*-value of 0.003 (Figure 6.6a). While neither the null nor the alternative hypothesis regarding the high-dose cisplatin plus mitomycin-C arm could be rejected, the rationale for the use of high-dose

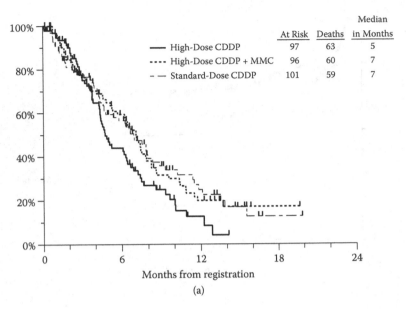

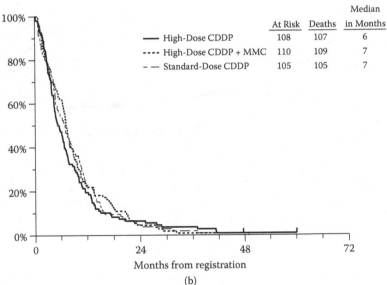

FIGURE 6.6
Survival in SWOG lung cancer trial 8738: (a) at time of closure; (b) at time of publication.

cisplatin, with or without mitomycin-C, had been called into question. Furthermore, the two high-dose arms had significantly more toxicity than the standard-dose arm. The monitoring committee decided the whole trial should be closed at this point. At the time of publication the results were still negative (Figure 6.6b).

6.6.1.3 Stopping an Equivalence Trial Early for Positive Results

SWOG study S8412 (Alberts et al., 1992) was designed to test "equivalence" of IV cisplatin + cyclophosphamide versus IV carboplatin + cyclophosphamide in stage III-IV ovarian cancer. Early experience with carboplatin suggested it was substantially less toxic than its analog cisplatin, so the goal of the trial was to demonstrate that cisplatin's antitumor effects were not substantially superior. The null hypothesis was a 30% improvement due to cisplatin, and the trial was designed to have sufficient power to reject this hypothesis if the treatment arms were equivalent.

The first major decision of the monitoring committee for this trial was to consider a change of primary endpoint from pathologic complete response (CR) to survival. A problem with pathologic CR was that we weren't getting complete information. Too many patients with clinical CRs were not getting second-look surgeries, so pathologic CR could not be determined. Two patients with clinical evidence of disease had second look surgeries anyway (despite its not being required) and no disease was found. Both facts suggested an analysis based on pathologic CR would be biased. Furthermore, even if pathologic CR had been determined completely, differences would not necessarily imply patients were better or worse off long term. The change to survival was made and the stopping guidelines were modified accordingly.

At the time of the first formal interim analysis (at approximately 1/4 of the anticipated number of deaths), a 30% improvement in survival due to the cisplatin arm was ruled out at the specified level for early stopping; in fact, at this point the carboplatin arm appeared superior with respect to survival. The decision to stop the trial was not clear-cut, however. The apparent lack of survival benefit due to cisplatin and the clear superiority of carboplatin with respect to most of the severe cisplatin toxicities had to be weighed against an increase in thrombocytopenia on the carboplatin arm, inconclusive results with respect to response and time to failure, and no long-term survival information. Discussion in the monitoring committee included observations from investigators treating patients on the trial that they were relieved when their patients were randomized to carboplatin and so could expect less vomiting. Discussion also included thoughtful comments from the NCI representative concerning the risk of an equivocal trial after further follow-up if the study were closed early. A less helpful suggestion from some of the members was to report the trial but continue randomizing anyway. (This would have been contrary to the DMC policy of not reporting on active trials. It also seems inconsistent to conclude results are convincing enough to report but not to stop treating with the inferior agent.) After a formal meeting and two rounds of letters, it was decided that results were sufficiently convincing to stop accrual and to report the trial.

Figure 6.7a shows how results looked at the time we closed the trial and Figure 6.7b shows results at the time of publication. Results remained inconsistent with a 30% improvement due to cisplatin. Note the similarity to Figures 6.6a and b, which illustrate stopping for a negative result. In each case we were able to stop because the hypothesized better arm looked worse

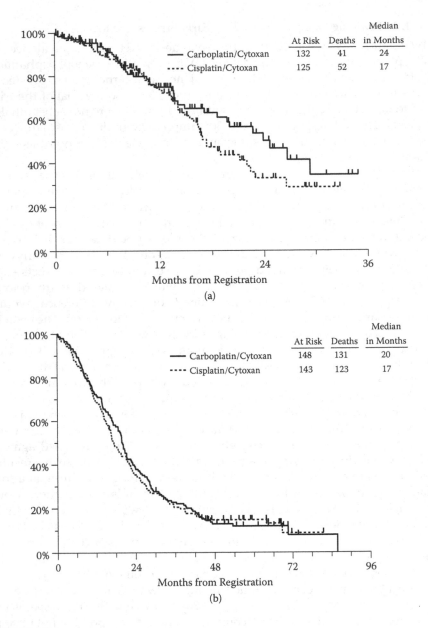

FIGURE 6.7
Survival in SWOG ovarian cancer trial 8412: (a) at time of closure; (b) at time of publication.

instead. The results most likely were exaggerated due to the random ups and downs that occur during the course of any trial, and in each study the difference decreased by the time of the final analysis. Results remained convincingly negative for each, however, due to the conservative approach to stopping.

6.6.1.4 Stopping Based on Toxicity and Lack of Compliance

Limited small-cell lung cancer study S8812 (Bunn et al., 1995; Kelly et al., 1995) was designed originally to test whether the addition of interferon to brain radiotherapy improved survival in responders to induction therapy. Formal interim analyses were to be performed after approximately 400 and 600 responders had been accrued. A secondary goal was added in protocol development, to determine if a decrease in the number of severe infections in patients receiving induction therapy (RT plus concurrent VP-16 and cis-platin) could be accomplished by adding GM-CSF to stimulate granulocyte production. The early stopping guideline for this endpoint called for an interim analysis after 160 patients had been evaluated for infection; the final analysis for this endpoint was to be done after 350 patients.

The induction chemotherapy used on this trial was a regimen from a pilot study with some minor modifications. Modifications included dropping vincristine, changing agents for the final cycles of treatment, modification of doses, different days of administration and a different retreatment interval. Any one of these might have been minor; all together they turned out not to be. In retrospect a new pilot study would have been prudent. Trouble was evident early. Five months after opening the study was temporarily closed due to severe hematologic toxicity. It was reopened 2 months later with reduced doses of chemotherapy. Severe toxicities were reduced but not eliminated, and it started to become clear that GM-CSF was causing some of the problems.

The monitoring committee had been reviewing information regularly. Emergency early closure was not necessary, but by the time of the interim analysis for the infection endpoint, results were clear. There was an unanticipated and striking increase in the number of patients with grade 4 thrombocytopenia on the GM-CSF arm (Table 6.12). There was also a possible increase in the number of severe infections, despite a small decrease in granulocytopenia (although this may have been due in part to misdiagnosis of radiation pneumonitis). The GM-CSF arm was closed.

Accrual to the no GM-CSF arm and randomization to maintenance were continued for another 6 months. At this time the monitoring committee closed the rest of the trial with only 125 on the maintenance randomization due to severe compliance problems. One-half of all patients on interferon were refusing therapy before relapse despite only moderate toxicity. The question

TABLE 6.12

Adverse Hematologic Events by Treatment Arm from SWOG S8812

	No GM-CSF	GM-CSF
Grade 4 granulocytopenia	19%	14%
Grade 4 leukopenia	11%	10%
Grade 4 thrombocytopenia	4%	30%
Fatal infection	0%	4%

of whether survival was improved by patients taking interferon as long as they could stand it was not considered of sufficient interest to continue the trial.

6.6.1.5 Emergency Stopping Based on Unexpected Toxic Deaths

One of the mechanisms of tumor resistance to therapy is thought to be development of a multidrug resistant tumor phenotype (specifically, expression of p-glycoprotein, a membrane protein involved in the transport of toxins from cells). Study S9028 (Salmon et al., 1998) was designed to test the hypothesis that standard therapy plus agents to block transport of drugs from cells would be more effective than standard therapy alone in the treatment of multiple myeloma. Patients were randomized to receive either vincristine, doxorubicin and dexamethasone (VAD) or VAD + verapamil and quinine (VQ) to overcome multidrug resistance.

A difficulty in evaluation of multiple myeloma patients is determination of cause of death. Patients who die due to disease often die of multiple organ (renal, cardiac, pulmonary, hematologic) failure, which makes it difficult to distinguish death due to disease from death due to various organ toxicities. SWOG S9028 opened to accrual on October 1, 1990, and several deaths of patients on VAD + VQ were reported to the statistical center over the summer of 1991. The Study Coordinator reviewed the charts and judged that these deaths, primarily due to renal failure in patients with poor renal function at diagnosis, were possibly related to verapamil. An amendment was prepared to reduce the dose of verapamil in these poor risk patients, and the data monitoring committee was notified of this action. By the time the committee met, in late October, the evidence implicating verapamil was more clear, though the survival difference was not statistically significant, and the VAD + VQ arm was closed to further accrual. Patients still being treated with VAD + VQ were switched from sustained action to standard formulation verapamil in December, following a report implicating the sustained action formulation (Pritza et al., 1991). After further deliberation by the investigators, all patients were taken off verapamil in February of 1992.

Clearly some things won't wait for a semi-annual meeting of a data monitoring committee. The data monitoring committee was important in agreeing previous actions were appropriate and in recommending further action, but if statistical center staff and the study coordinator had waited to do evaluations until it was time for the data monitoring committee to meet, other patients on this trial would likely have died toxic deaths. Could actions have been taken even sooner? We have all spent time worrying about this, but think the answer is probably "not much sooner." The initial deaths looked like typical myeloma deaths so earlier detection of the problem was not likely. The excess of deaths in poor risk patients was alarming, but the difference between the arms could have been due to chance. Since the study hypothesis was still sound, a first approach of reducing the verapamil dose in poor risk patients seemed justified. Perhaps the dates for discontinuing accrual, changing to standard formula, and of dropping verapamil altogether could have been earlier—but not early enough to have changed the management of any of the patients who died.

6.6.1.6 Concluding Remarks on Interim Analyses

No method of interim analysis works if an extra analysis is done because results look interesting. "Looks interesting/doesn't look interesting" amounts to an interim analysis in itself. If this is done repeatedly with the possibility of a formal test each time (whether or not the test is done), the number of interim analysis times becomes far greater than the number specified in the design. All of the careful probability calculations used to specify multistage designs are based on the assumption that analysis is independent of outcome.

6.7 Phase II/III Trials

Phase II/III trials provide a mechanism for reducing the development time due to waiting for Phase II results before designing and launching the subsequent Phase III trial. In one class of Phase II/III designs, multiple experimental arms and a control arm are randomized, with an early (Phase II) look either to stop the trial or continue with fewer arms. One or more of the candidates are selected at an early analysis (Phase II part) for continued randomization and full Phase III comparison, generally based on meeting a threshold difference versus control. Final testing is adjusted for the tests used in the interim selection procedure. Thall et al. (1988) address this approach when the primary endpoint is binomial, while Schaid et al. (1990) address the time-to-event case. Royston et al. (2003) propose eliminating unpromising arms early using a short-term endpoint, and combine information from the Phase II and Phase III portions by modeling the relationship between the short-term and the primary long-term endpoint. Stallard and Todd (2003) formulate the problem more generally using an approach that allows for additional interim analyses after the Phase II screening analysis (see also Bauer and Kieser (1999)). In a variation on the theme, Liu and Pledger (2005) describe an approach to screening dose levels using a short-term endpoint for initial (Phase II) testing before completion of a Phase III of remaining dose levels vs control with the longer-term endpoint. In this design, patients continue to be accrued to all doses during collection of the early endpoints in first stage patients. After the first stage short-term endpoint information is complete, doses are chosen and accrual is discontinued to arms that lack efficacy or cause safety concerns. The final test of experimental dose d is a weighted average of a test of control versus dose d in first stage patients and a test for dose d in the second stage patients, both with respect to the longer term endpoint.

Issues in using these approaches include the complexity of the statistical considerations, for instance, the choice of level and power. Typical choices for level are (1) the probability of concluding at least one arm effective given all arms are equal or (2) the level for each pairwise comparison adjusted for multiple comparisons. Power is often defined as either the probability of concluding the correct arm is superior to control under a least favorable alternative or as the pairwise power. Considerable effort is needed to design trials to have properties that suit each clinical setting. Another issue is that the initial screening procedure will not always work well. For instance if a procedure chooses only one arm, then when more than one arm is effective, one will likely be chosen but not necessarily the best arm—the relatively small sample sizes at the screening look do not allow for accurate distinction between arms with moderate differences. In addition, the Phase III part of such trials will be larger than a stand-alone Phase III due to the initial testing. A final issue is that these types of studies can be operationally difficult to manage, as they may involve temporarily stopping the trial, changes in case report forms, protocol amendments, addition of participating sites, and re-review by Institutional Review Boards.

As discussed in Chapter 5, there is an increasing trend toward the use of randomized Phase II trials, especially with primary endpoints other than response, and with subsets defined by the presence of molecular targets. These factors make reliance on historical controls, even for Phase II trials, problematic. However, there is some concern that trials designed merely to *lead* to definitive Phase III comparisons will instead be ends in themselves, as results from small randomized trials are published and then treated as more convincing than intended (Redman and Crowley, 2007). To address this concern, and in an effort to streamline the overall drug development process, several two arm Phase II/III designs have been proposed. Most of these involve modeling the relationship between shorter-term outcomes appropriate for Phase II trials, such as response and progression-free survival, and longer-term outcomes typical of Phase III trials, such as overall survival, as done by Royston et al.

An early proposal along these lines, dubbed a "seamless" Phase II/III trial, is due to Inoue et al. (2002), who used a Bayesian approach to modeling the relationship between response and survival in the context of non-small cell lung cancer. The Phase II portion of their proposal was based on response and was for a limited number of institutions, while the Phase III portion was based on survival and an expanded set of institutions. Simulations demonstrated the efficiency of this approach, compared to separate sequential Phase II and then Phase III trials, in terms of the total number of patients required for given error rates.

A more traditional approach to this problem was proposed and investigated by Hunsberger et al. (2009). They suggest formally embedding the randomized Phase II trial, as described for example by Rubinstein et al., 2005, based on progression-free survival, into a Phase III trial with overall survival as the primary endpoint. The first interim analysis for this Phase II/III trial is thus a go/no go decision based on rejecting/not rejecting the null hypothesis using the Type I error rate appropriate for a randomized Phase II trial (one-sided Type I error rate of 0.10–0.20). If the decision is to proceed, the Phase II patients are used in further interim and final analyses based on survival. They show by simulation that considerable savings in total sample size are possible, compared to sequential Phase II (either single arm or randomized) and Phase III trials, or a single Phase III trial based on survival, for given probabilities of drawing false positive or negative conclusions. A large part of the savings comes from using progression-free survival as the endpoint for the Phase II portion, as opposed to using overall survival at the first interim analysis, as previously noted by Goldman et al. (2008).

SWOG has recently proposed just such a Phase II/III trial, for the first line treatment of patients with small-cell lung cancer. The standard of therapy is cisplatin/etoposide, and the experimental arm adds the new agent cediranib. The first interim analysis is to be a randomized Phase II trial with one-sided Type I error 0.15 and power 0.90 for an alternative hypothesis of a 70% increase in median progression-free survival. The sample size for this portion of the trial is $N = 198$, assuming that there is to be no temporary closure for additional follow-up after the Phase II portion. Only if this is positive (null hypothesis of no difference is rejected) will the trial proceed. Subsequent interim and final analyses are based on survival, with an alternative hypothesis of a 40% increase in median survival. The final analysis uses a one-sided Type I error of 0.02. The total (maximum) sample size is $N = 576$, and the overall power is 0.86. A stand-alone randomized Phase II trial of 198 patients, followed by a typical Phase III trial, would require $198 + 480 = 678$ to achieve the same statistical properties as the proposed Phase II/III design. With the usual follow-up for events after accrual to a Phase II trial, however, only 150 patients would be required, or $150 + 480 = 630$ total for the sequential trials, as opposed to 576 for the Phase II/III trial. An important point for this approach is that the power for the first portion needs to be higher than for the usual randomized Phase II trial, e.g., 90%, for the overall power of the trial to be reasonable, since this will be a product of the Phase II power and the conditional power for the remainder of the trial, given a positive result from the Phase II portion at the first interim analysis.

6.8 Concluding Remark

Much recent work has been done on "adaptive designs." Adaptive design may be defined as "a clinical study design that uses accumulating data to decide how to modify aspects of the study as it continues, without undermining the validity and integrity of the trial" (Gallo et al., 2006). This designation applies to many types of designs, including the designs described in Section 6.6 (group sequential designs for interim monitoring and sample size re-estimation designs), and the designs described in 6.7 (multi-arm designs that drop less promising regimens before continuing to a definitive Phase III, designs that model the relationship of early and late endpoints as the trial progresses, and designs that incorporate Phase II and Phase III testing into a single randomized study). Benefits in terms of efficiency are possible using these designs, although these benefits are often accompanied by longer development time due to technical and computational complications, greater operational challenges and additional risks for non-definitive results due to the additional assumptions needed for the designs.

7

Data Management and Quality Control

The quality of the data never stopped me from doing a quality analysis.

—(Quote from a famous statistician. We think it best not to say which one.)

7.1 Introduction: Why Worry?

As the old adage goes, garbage in, garbage out. Simply put, faulty data compromise studies. Survival estimates are biased if patients are lost to follow-up; early results are biased by inclusion of patients who will later be found to be ineligible and by missing information; response estimates are biased if tumor assessments are missed; variability is increased if patients are not treated according to protocol, making it more difficult to detect treatment differences. The following three examples are illustrative.

Figure 7.1 shows the Kaplan-Meier estimate of survival from a sample of 10 patients, five of whom have been lost to follow-up. The lost patients are censored at the time they were last known to be alive. The bottom curve shows the estimate for the extreme in which all five lost patients died right after being lost; while the top curve shows the extreme in which all lost patients actually survived until the time of analysis at 4 years. The survival estimate will be biased high if patients were lost because they were beginning to fail, and it will be biased low if patients were lost because they were doing well. Both scenarios are plausible: Patients on advanced disease studies may go elsewhere if they aren't doing well; patients on early stage studies who remain disease-free for many years may stop showing up for appointments.

Figures 7.2 through 7.4 illustrate with a real example how results change when the data are cleaned up. A SWOG study compared CMFVP with L-PAM (L-phenylalanine mustard, or melphalan) as adjuvant treatment in resectable node-positive breast cancer (Rivkin et al., 1989). Initially a significant difference was observed in postmenopausal patients, with logrank $p = 0.003$, as shown in Figure 7.2. After cleaning up the data with respect to eligibility and unrecorded events, this difference decreased, with the logrank p-value changing to 0.08 (Figure 7.3). After a request for updated follow-up, the difference decreased more, with a p-value of 0.17 (Figure 7.4). The example illustrates how uncorrected data can be misleading.

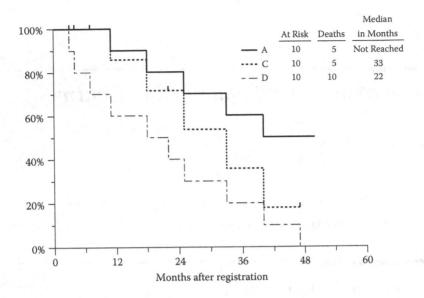

FIGURE 7.1
Potential bias in estimates where five patients have been lost to follow-up. Curve A: assumed alive. Curve C: censored. Curve D: assumed dead.

As a final example of how faulty data can bias results, consider the following scenario. A patient enters on study with a 2.0-cm lung lesion on computed tomography (CT) and a positive bone scan. At the first two assessments after entry the lung lesion is 0.5 cm; at the second a bone scan is also done, as required, and shows no change. At the third assessment the lesion is 1.5 cm.

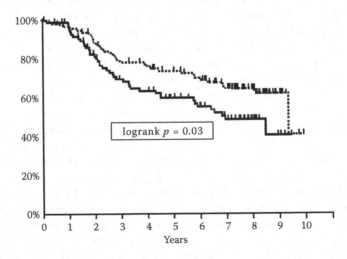

FIGURE 7.2
Survival distributions before data cleanup, and with follow-up overdue.

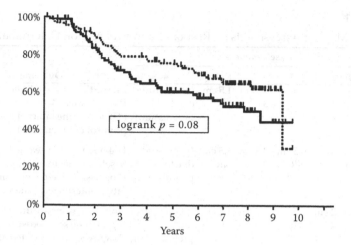

FIGURE 7.3
Survival distributions after data cleanup, and with follow-up overdue.

Using RECIST v1.1 response criteria, the patient has a partial response starting at the first assessment, the response is confirmed at a second assessment, and progression of disease occurs at the time of the third assessment. (Note that while this 1.5 cm lesion is still smaller than the original 2.0 cm lesion, it represents a tripling over the minimum measurements at the second and third assessments, and is thus defined as a progression.) Table 7.1 shows what happens if tests are missed. If assessment 1 or 2 is missed or done differently, the response is either unconfirmed or missed altogether. If assessment 3 is

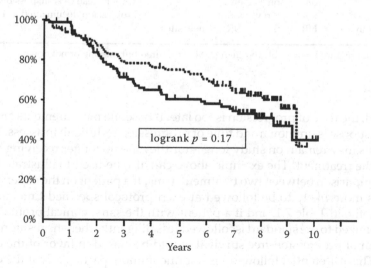

FIGURE 7.4
Survival distributions after data cleanup, and with follow-up updated.

TABLE 7.1

Effect of Missing Assessments on Response and Progression Determination*

		Assessment				
	Baseline	1	2	3	4	Outcome
Lung scan	2 cm	0.5 cm	0.5 cm	1.5 cm	(pt off study	PR starting at 1, confirmed at 2
Bone scan	+	NR	S	NR	due to	Progression at 3
					progression)	("Truth" to the limits of the protocol requirements.)
Lung scan	M	0.5 cm	0.5 cm	1.5 cm	(pt off study	Unknown response due to no
Bone scan	+	NR	S	NR	due to	baseline measurement
					progression)	Progression documented at 3 (at 1 if interpreted as new lesion)
Lung scan	2 cm	0.5 cm	0.5 cm	1.5 cm	(pt off study	Unknown response due to no
Bone scan	+	NR	M	M	due to	repeat bone scan; possible PR
					progression)	Progression documented at 3
Lung scan	2 cm	0.5 cm	M	1.5 cm	(pt off study	PR starting at 1, not confirmed
Bone scan	+	NR	S	NR	due to	Progression documented at 3
					progression)	
Lung scan	2 cm	M	M	1.5 cm	2.2 cm	PR starting at 3, not confirmed
Bone scan	+	NR	M	S	new sites	Progression documented at 4
Lung scan	2 cm	M	0.5 cm	M	2.2 cm	PR starting at 2, not confirmed
Bone scan	+	NR	S	NR	new sites	Stable at 3, progression documented at 4
Lung scan	2 cm	M	M	M	2.2 cm	???? No response, unknown if
Bone scan	M	M	M	M	+	progression, patient continued on treatment
Lung scan	2 cm	1.5 cm on x-ray	1.5 cm on x-ray	2 cm on x-ray	2.2 cm	Unknown response due to x-ray instead of scan; possibly stable Progression documented at 4
Bone scan	+	NR	S	NR	new sites	

*NR = not required, S = stable/no change, M = required but missing or not done.

missed, the time of progression is too late. If baseline measurements are missing, response is unknown and time of progression is difficult to assess. Worse, patients may remain on study long after they are no longer receiving benefit from the treatment. The example above can also be used to illustrate bias in the comparison between two treatment arms. If a patient on the experimental arm is more likely to be followed at each protocol specified time, and has the profile in Table 7.1, and if a patient with the same clinical profile who is randomized to the standard is followed less diligently, then the resulting comparison of progression-free survival would be biased in favor of the control arm. This differential follow-up is not uncommon, particularly if the control arm is an observation arm, or if the control has a well-known and tolerated toxicity profile.

The rest of this chapter describes some of the ways to maintain quality data, from protocol development through data collection and evaluation procedures. Experiences are described from the point of view of a multi-institutional, multi-study organization, a setting in which it is most difficult to maintain consistency and quality.

7.2 Protocol Development

The protocol document sets the standards by which the study will be conducted. A clearly written and well-justified protocol document is a critical early step in the conduct of good quality clinical trials. While there are many formats that produce successful protocols, it is important that the protocol document include explicit information on the topics presented below. Using a standard format is helpful in various ways. It allows for ease of reference by the institutions that have to use the protocol, for streamlining of production of the document, and for interpretation of the same items in the same way across protocols. It also allows for consistent inclusion of important aspects in the protocol, and for automatic clarification of common problems. During the process of developing the protocol, different parties may be responsible for drafting different sections, but all study team members should review the protocol carefully for consistency, for clarity of instructions, correctness of procedures and feasibility of the objectives. The following sections appear in all SWOG protocol documents. SWOG study S8811 (Margolin et al., 1994), which was a Phase II study of 5-FU with continuous infusion of high-dose folinic acid in advanced breast cancer, is used to illustrate.

7.2.1 Objectives

This section should include all primary and secondary objectives, and each should be explicitly defined. It is not sufficient, for example, to state that a goal is "to assess the use of adjuvant chemo-radiation in the treatment of gastric cancer." Instead, the primary goal should be stated as "to compare survival of gastric cancer patients treated with chemo-radiation following surgery to those treated with surgery alone." For S8811, the primary objective was to assess response to 5-FU and folinic acid as treatment for advanced breast cancer, in order to decide whether the regimen should be tested further. Secondary objectives also specified were to assess toxicity and survival for patients treated with this regimen.

7.2.2 Background

The background provides justification for addressing the objectives. The background in the protocol for S8811 included both biologic rationale and clinical observations. Biologically, it was hypothesized that folinic acid enhanced the activity of 5-FU by potentiating the inhibition of thymidylate synthetase. If true, then addition of folinic acid to 5-FU would be expected to improve the antitumor effect of 5-FU. The clinical observations supporting study of the regimen included an estimated response probability of 0.17 in a group of heavily pretreated patients, most of whom had previously failed on standard 5-FU therapy. The background also included information on response to standard 5-FU, which was necessary in order to justify the assumptions used in developing the statistical considerations.

7.2.3 Drug Information

This section should be standardized so that all protocols with the same agent have consistent information provided. Sections on new routes or agents can be obtained from the National Cancer Institute, if it is an NCI-supplied agent. Chemistry, toxicology, and pharmaceutical data are described in this section and the supplier is specified. Having standardized drug descriptions aids in efficient production of the protocol and avoids conflicting information across protocols.

7.2.4 Stage Definitions

Applicable disease-specific stage definitions should be standard if at all possible. There are standard definitions for most cancers, typically based on the American Joint Commission on Cancer staging definitions (Edge et al., 2010). This section may not be applicable for some diseases.

7.2.5 Eligibility Criteria

Eligibility criteria typically cover disease characteristics, prior treatment, and patient characteristics. These criteria should describe the patients to whom the results of the trial are to be generalized, and should be limited to only those requirements which are absolutely necessary. For S8811, disease requirements included adenocarcinoma of the breast, and measurable metastatic or recurrent disease. For prior treatment requirements, patients must have had no more than one prior chemotherapy for metastatic disease. Required patient characteristics included pretreatment WBC above 4000, platelets above 150,000, creatinine and bilirubin less than 1.5 times the upper limit of normal (ULN), and patients had to be ambulatory. The standard regulatory requirements concerned pregnancy (which was not allowed), Institutional Review Board approval (which had to be current), and informed consent (which had to be signed by the patient prior to registration). Careful attention to the eligibility sections when the protocol is developed saves a lot of trouble later. If the criteria are unclear, then there will not be a clearly defined patient population that can be precisely described in the manuscript. There will be misunderstandings by the participating institutions, resulting in too many ineligible patients being registered. There will be protocol revisions to be written and circulated. A clear and precise eligibility section is particularly important when there is a policy not to allow exceptions to the criteria—which there should be if the study is to be credible. For instance, if WBC greater than 4000 is required, then a patient with a WBC equal to or below 4000 can't be accepted. Criteria that are not meant to be enforced should not be in the eligibility section of the protocol. One alternative to making exact lab value comparisons is to instead require that the patient be healthy enough for protocol treatment according to good medical practices.

SWOG organizes the eligibility criteria by listing all the inclusion criteria first (the patient must have these), followed by the exclusion criterion (the patient must not have these). It may be helpful to include all information about a particular requirement in one, and only one criteria. For example, requiring a white blood cell count of at least 4000 can be stated as an inclusion criterion, or disallowing a white blood cell less than 4000 can be stated as an exclusion criterion, but both are not necessary.

7.2.6 Stratification Factors and Subsets

Stratification factors are used in the study design to allocate patients to treatment on randomized studies (see Chapter 6 for a discussion of stratification factors). Subsets are those factors for which separate accrual goals and separate analyses are specified. Most Phase II studies do not have stratification factors or subsets. In S8811, however, there was interest in answering questions in two separate types of patients, so there was one subset factor. Patients were accrued separately into two groups: one with no prior chemotherapy for advanced disease and one with one prior chemotherapy.

7.2.7 Treatment Plan

This section contains a detailed treatment plan, including a table that details dose level, route of administration, days of treatment, retreatment interval and the order of the different agents. A sample treatment table is included at the end of this chapter. This section of the protocol also specifies any restrictions on ancillary treatment. Typically concurrent cancer treatment is not allowed so that outcomes can be attributed to the treatment under study. There may also be supportive care treatments that are preferred (e.g., a particular antiemetic regimen) or contraindicated (e.g., no corticosteroids), or guidelines for use of growth factors or antibiotics. The section also provides a list of acceptable reasons for removal of a patient from treatment.

7.2.8 Treatment Modification

This section gives detailed instructions for treatment modification if the patient experiences excessive toxicity. The section includes the phone number of the study coordinator and a back-up clinician for institutions to contact with any questions concerning problems with treatment. These questions should not be left to a clinical research associate at the institution or to the study management personnel—it is inappropriate for them to give medical advice, even if what seems to be the same question is raised over and over.

It is important that the treatment and dose modification sections be clear, not only for the safety of the patients, but also for consistency. If instructions aren't clear, patients will be treated in a variety of different ways. For instance, suppose the protocol says "decrease dose by 25% after a one week delay if the patient experiences grade 3 vomiting." Does this mean to decrease by 25% of the starting dose or of the previous dose? If it means the starting dose and the patient experiences grade 3 vomiting a second time, does the patient stay at 75% starting dose, or is dose reduced by another 25% of starting dose? Should the dose be escalated back to starting dose if the patient recovers? What if the patient is still vomiting after one week? Obscure instructions will add variability to the study and may compromise its interpretation.

7.2.9 Study Calendar

The study calendar specifies all baseline tests and the schedule for all follow-up tests that are required for eligibility, disease assessment, and adverse event assessment. It also specifies the follow-up schedule after a patient goes off treatment. The calendar helps ensure patients are uniformly and correctly assessed. Check to be sure the baseline requirements include everything needed to determine eligibility and the follow-up requirements include everything needed to assess adverse events and disease. Omit any test not required. For instance, alkaline phosphatase might be fairly routine, but if not necessary for an adequate assessment, leave it to the discretion of the individual investigators. Also be sure to qualify requirements as appropriate. For instance, compliance with an unqualified requirement for a pregnancy test or for monthly CT scans is likely to be poor.

7.2.10 Endpoint Definitions

Endpoint definitions generally include response, performance status, survival, and progression-free survival or time to treatment failure. SWOG uses endpoint definitions that are consistent across protocols. For instance, all studies have the same definition of survival and performance status, and all solid tumor studies have the same definition of response. Clear definitions are needed so that endpoints are interpreted the same way at each institution. (Some of the difficulties in defining endpoints are discussed in Chapter 3.) Errors are avoided if the definitions are detailed and if the same definitions are always used. If there isn't consistency, it becomes difficult for institutions to keep track of and apply many different definitions across many different protocols. It also becomes difficult to interpret manuscripts when the same endpoint (nominally) always means something different.

7.2.11 Statistical Considerations

How statistical considerations are produced is covered in Chapters 2–6. In general, this section includes accrual estimates, sample size with justification, study duration, and a specification of the types of interim and final analyses to be performed. With respect to study quality, the point to make is that what is written in the statistical considerations should be consistent with the rest of the protocol, particularly with respect to the objectives and the background.

7.2.12 Discipline Review

Special reviews of pathology, radiation therapy, and surgery are done when quality control of these is important on a study. For example, radiation therapy typically should be reviewed if the procedures are nonstandard and an important part of protocol treatment. Surgery should be reviewed under the same circumstances, or if it is part of disease assessment, such as confirming a pathologic complete response. Reviews are probably too expensive to justify if the procedures are routine. For instance, SWOG does not review mastectomies done prior to registration on adjuvant breast cancer studies. Reviews were done at one time, but 287 reviews resulted in only one patient found to be ineligible solely as a consequence of surgical review; it was judged not worth the effort to continue routine review. On the other hand, surgical review of second look surgeries is often important in ovarian cancer studies.

Pathology should be reviewed if there is moderate difficulty in making a pathologic diagnosis. If there is little difficulty, the effort it takes to review slides is greater than the gain. If there is a great deal of difficulty, it's also probably not worth it, unless one of the specific aims of the study is to study pathology.

For all of the disciplines, standard submission procedures should be used whenever possible. Limiting the number of routines the institutions have to follow results in fewer mistakes.

7.2.13 Registration Instructions

In addition to the method(s) of registration available to participating institutions, this section reminds institutions of three registration policies. First, registrations after treatment start are not allowed; second, registrations cannot be canceled after they are completed; third, the planned treatment start date should be within 1 working day after registration for most studies.

The first two policies are in place to minimize biases that can occur when there are options to include or exclude patients as a function of how well they are doing or as a function of which arm was assigned. If patients who have already started treatment can be registered, only those who do not quit or fail right away will be entered, making the treatment look better than it is. If cancellations are allowed, then it is possible that patients will be followed on study only when they are randomized to the arm they wanted anyway, which defeats the purpose of randomization. A trial (not in SWOG) of surgery versus radiation therapy in prostate cancer had to be abandoned for just this reason. Each patient received the assigned treatment if it was the one their clinician wanted them to get, and was omitted from the registration list if not—so patients received exactly the same treatments they would have without randomization, thereby reducing the trial to an observational study.

The third policy is enforced in order to minimize the number of patients who do not receive treatment. If long delays between registration and treatment start are allowed, some patients will deteriorate and no longer be candidates for treatment, some will die, and others will change their minds and refuse assigned treatment. Since all eligible patients who are registered on study must be used in the analysis of the study (see Chapter 8), it is best to have as few of these cases as possible.

7.2.14 Data Submission Instructions

The data submission instructions include which case report forms are required, the time limits for CRF submission, and instructions for submission. For adequate monitoring, time limits for data submission after registration, discontinuation of treatment, progression of disease, and death are short (7–14 days from the event for most studies).

7.2.15 Special Instructions

A special instructions section is important for extra study-specific requirements that do not warrant an explicit section elsewhere in the protocol. For example, this section might include specimen submission instructions for biologic studies, or instruction on how to administer questionnaires for quality of life endpoints.

7.2.16 Regulatory Requirements

Regulatory requirements can include instructions for reporting serious adverse events (SAEs), and an outline of informed consent requirements.

7.2.17 Bibliography

This section contains the bibliography of references.

7.2.18 Forms

Forms to be used in the study are included in Section 18. Forms are discussed below.

7.2.19 Appendix

The appendices can include data reporting requirements, such as adverse event criteria. As of this printing, the Common Terminology Criteria for Adverse Events (CTCAE) version 4.0 is the most recent standard set forth by the National Cancer Institute for reporting adverse events. Clinical research associates are expected to report adverse events using these terms and grade definitions, which helps consistency of interpretation across protocols. The CTCAE is updated approximately every two years, and can be mapped to the Medical Dictionary for Regulatory Activities (MedDRA).

7.3 Data Collection

The development and conduct of a clinical trial is an expensive proposition, not only in dollars, but in terms of patient resources and researcher time. It is tempting to collect as much data as possible in hopes of maximizing the returns on any trial. Unfortunately, this strategy is likely to backfire. Anyone who has participated in a survey is familiar with the change from initial enthusiasm to tedium and impatience that accompanies the progression through completion of a lengthy questionnaire. There is a similar effect in data collection for clinical research. The quality of what is collected is inversely related to the quantity of information requested. A researcher will be more likely to take care to provide accurate information on five items, but is less likely to take the same care with a list of 50 data items. As a result, a manuscript based on a small number of carefully reported variables will be limited, but correct, whereas the second scenario yields a manuscript that will be extensive, but less accurate, or possibly not worth writing at all. Even when the quantity of data is limited, care must be taken to ensure that data are well defined, and reporting carefully controlled.

To achieve the goal of maximizing the accuracy of information reported on a trial, collection should be limited to those data crucial to the main goals of the trial. As data collection plans are developed, proposed variables should be included if they fall into one of the following categories:

1. needed to support a specific aim of the study;
2. required to properly stratify a patient;
3. recognized as prognostic variables necessary for analysis;
4. required to document patient eligibility;
5. required to guarantee patient safety;
6. mandated for reporting purposes (e.g., race, method of payment are variables required by the National Cancer Institute).

Collection of any variables that do not fall into one of the above categories should be severely limited.

In the following sections we outline data collection strategies followed by SWOG. While many of the discussions are specific to cancer research in a Cooperative Group, the principles remain the same in any clinical research setting.

7.3.1 Basic Data Items

A key way that SWOG has standardized study conduct has been to define a fixed set of data items used for all treatment studies. This has been very important for data management and quality control. It allows for uniform training of data coordinators and study coordinators, for consistency of inter-pretation of variables across all disease sites, and it allows for extensive logic checks to be developed for application to all studies.

Our set of standard variables fall into four groups: eligibility, evaluabil-ity, treatment summary, and outcome summary. Various considerations went into the development of the set. We weighed the cost of collecting an item of information against its usefulness. For instance, collecting quality of life in-formation is very expensive (Moinpour, 1996) and compliance is often poor; thus quality of life is not part of our standard outcome data set. Another example is calculation of dose received. This is also very time consuming and, particularly in the case of oral drugs, inaccurate. Furthermore, analy-sis by dose received is fatally flawed (see Chapter 9), so the primary use for the effort is a single line in a manuscript giving a (poor) estimate of how much of the planned drug the patients received. There are some studies where this may be sufficiently important (studies designed to investigate dose intensity questions) to make received dose calculations a priority, but not enough studies to make this part of our standard data set. Our basic treatment items consist of start and stop dates and treatment status, which indicates whether or not the patient is on protocol treatment, and if not, the reason why not. We also code a crude summary of amount of treatment re-ceived (none, minimal, or more than minimal where the definition of minimal can be treatment-specific), and we also code whether or not there was a major deviation. Major deviations are reserved for gross treatment violations, such as no treatment given or the wrong treatment arm given or a major dosing error.

Another principle we followed in developing the basic data set was not to mix up different concepts, or to have items where more than one answer would apply. For instance, a previous version of SWOG evaluation variables included an item that combined eligibility, evaluability, major treatment de-viations and reason off treatment; the choices were: (1) ineligible; (2) fully evaluable; (3) partially evaluable due to refusal; (4) partially evaluable due to toxicity; (5) partially evaluable due to early death; (6) partially evaluable due to other reasons; (7) lost to follow-up; (8) not evaluable due to major violation; (9) not evaluable due to insufficient information; or (10) not evalu-able due to other reasons. Since only one could be chosen, even though several could apply, the variable was inadequate for summarizing basic information needed for manuscripts—e.g., it couldn't be assumed that the number of patients lost to follow-up was the same as the number of patients coded "7."

In addition to cost and logic, a third consideration in defining the standard data set was to minimize what we asked for, as discussed above. This principle was implemented in two ways. The standard data set includes key variables that are collected on all patients, regardless of disease type. Additionally, each disease committee identified a limited standard set of basic data that are collected for all studies of a specific disease and stage type. Thus, for example, all studies of patients with metastatic colorectal cancer will collect a small basic set of variables that define the sites and characteristics of the disease. In addition to guaranteeing that the most important variables are collected, this ensures consistent coding of variables across studies. Study specific items may need to be added, but are also kept to a minimum.

The proper balance on detail can be difficult to judge. For instance, evaluability can be particularly difficult to define. All patients entered on a study are evaluable to some extent, but the extent can vary considerably—a simple yes-no or even yes-partial-no doesn't cover enough of the possibilities. We decided to record information on baseline disease status (measurable disease, evaluable disease, non-evaluable disease, no evidence of disease, or incomplete assessment of baseline status). For evaluability after the patient is on study we have one item that indicates whether or not the patient was assessed for adverse events and, if so, the date of last adverse event assessment, plus items that indicate whether the patient had disease assessment adequate for determining response and time to progression. These are all coded regardless of the eligibility of the patient—which brings us to the next example. The most basic eligibility variable would be a simple yes or no, but it may be worthwhile to keep some additional detail in order to be able to assess where problems are and address them. If patients are being found ineligible based on discipline review only, then perhaps educational sessions on what constitutes proper surgery, or on how to interpret histologic criteria might be in order. If patients are being found ineligible because of inadequate documentation, then perhaps submission procedures need to be tightened up. If ineligibility occurs because investigators ignore the criteria, then perhaps the investigators should be replaced.

A fourth consideration in defining our standard data items was completeness. Response is an example—the set "complete response, partial response, stable, increasing disease" is incomplete because too often tumor assessments are insufficient to determine response. When that happens, we use one of the following: "early death" is coded if the patient dies before disease can be assessed and death cannot be assumed due to disease, "unconfirmed response" is coded if there is only one assessment documenting response and "no assessment" is coded if assessments are missing and there is insufficient information to determine best response.

Although the primary point of this section is the importance of standardization when many studies are being done by many institutions, the considerations for developing a standard data set are the same for the single institution/single study setting as well. Cost/benefit of items, separate items for different concepts, number of items limited to a number that can be collected accurately, and logical completeness will still be key.

7.3.2 Case Report Form Design

A dream of many of those involved in the conduct of clinical trials is that the day will come when all the data needed to analyze a study have already been captured in the hospital information system or computerized medical record and merely need to be transmitted to a research database and summarized. That day is still a long way off. If everyone agreed to use compatible hardware and software the technological hurdles would not be particularly hard to overcome, but the universal experience to date is that data collected for one purpose (such as patient care) are not suitable for another (such as clinical research). The requisite data either are not available, are not coded appropriately, or are not of sufficient quality. Thus research data must be culled by skilled clinical research associates (CRAs) from several sources, some computerized and some not, and put into shape for transmission to the central statistical center. This is where the well-designed and easily understood case report form (CRF) comes in.

There are some very basic considerations that should be addressed when designing a case report form. Data items should follow standard naming conventions, so that it is clear what is being collected without the need for detailed instructions. A common standard in use for oncology trials is the Cancer Data Standards Repository (caDSR), which is maintained by the National Cancer Institute. Similar data items should be grouped together, so that they may be abstracted from single sections of the medical record. Data items that are conditional upon answers to other questions (e.g., "If Yes, then...") should be indented or otherwise formatted so that it is clear what conditions lead to the question. General form-specific instructions should be included to explain any difficult concepts, or include reminders about the submission schedule for the CRF.

It may be necessary to revise CRFs mid-study to add or remove data items, or to clarify instructions. The form version number or date should be included on the form, so that the CRA can be sure they are completing the correct one. Even when forms are to be submitted via electronic data capture systems (discussed below), CRAs may want to complete the form on paper first, and then transfer the data to the EDC system. So, a design that mimics the layout of a paper form can be helpful.

With respect to form content, most of the same considerations that go into developing a standardized data set go into the development of every form: standardizing where possible, weighing collection effort against usefulness (in this case the consideration is for collection effort at the institutions as opposed to effort in abstracting the standard data set from submitted information), restricting items on the form to ones that will be used (plus checking that no items that will be used are inadvertently left off), and making sure there are no logical difficulties in filling out the form.

SWOG routinely re-uses a set of standard CRFs. This includes an Off-Treatment Notice, Follow-up Form, and Notice of Death for almost all studies, and a Baseline Tumor Assessment and Follow-up Tumor Assessment form for solid tumor studies following response. The data items collected on these CRFs are broad enough to apply to a wide variety of studies. Some disease sites have other CRFs that can be used across studies within that disease. Re-using forms whenever possible increases familiarity and therefore accuracy from the CRAs completing them. CRFs that collect study-specific baseline, treatment, and adverse event data are typically created new for each SWOG study, but follow any standards that are in place for that disease site.

Baseline CRFs normally used on a SWOG study include a Prestudy form (also commonly referred to as an Onstudy form), Baseline Abnormalities form, and a Baseline Tumor Assessment form. The Prestudy form is a valuable instrument used to collect all items necessary to verify eligibility and stratification of the patient, as well as any important prognostic factors. The Baseline Abnormalities form collects detailed information about any pre-existing conditions which may affect the assessment of adverse events seen after protocol treatment begins. The Baseline Tumor Assessment form collects necessary information about the patient's disease status at the time of registration. This includes disease descriptions, tumor measurements, and assessment methods for comparison against later assessments.

Case report forms typically used to collect data while a patient is on protocol treatment include a Treatment form, an Adverse Event form, and a Follow-up Tumor Assessment form. The Treatment form collects any necessary information about the protocol treatment the patient received. This will include start and stop dates and dosing summary; concomitant medications and detailed lab data are only collected when necessary to meet a protocol objective. The Adverse Event form collects grades and for some studies, status (new versus continuing at the same grade versus worsening) of adverse events using the latest CTCAE definitions. The Follow-up Tumor Assessment form collects disease descriptions, tumor measurements, and assessment methods for the lesions identified on the Baseline Tumor Assessment form.

Once the patient is no longer receiving protocol treatment, an Off-Treatment Notice collects the summary of the treatment given, and the reason for discontinuation. Post-treatment follow-up data such as basic survival and disease assessment items are collected on the Follow-up form. If the patient should expire, data regarding the cause of death is collected on the Notice of Death.

For large studies, detailed treatment, adverse event and outcome information may be beyond the limit of what can be collected accurately. If the treatment regimens being used are not new, summary forms submitted once with simple treatment and adverse event information, plus follow-up forms asking for relapse and survival updates may be sufficient.

In order to maintain forms standards, new forms to be used in SWOG go through a review before implementation. A draft form is produced at the statistical center based on content proposed by the study coordinator and others who will be responsible for the conduct of the study, including the study statistician and the disease committee chair. The draft is reviewed and must be approved by these same people, plus a protocol review committee that consists of data coordinators and statisticians, plus database staff. If the forms are a significant departure from that to which institutions are accustomed, we also ask for comments from clinical research associates at the institutions. This process can be time consuming, but it is worthwhile in order to fix as many problems as possible before the forms are actually used in practice.

7.4 Data Submission

Many organizations, including SWOG, receive study data via electronic means, rather than on paper CRFs. Readily accessible high-speed Internet access in hospitals and clinics has made online data submission a viable alternative to a paper-based system. A lucrative industry now provides a wide variety of commercial electronic data capture (EDC) systems for collecting and managing clinical research data.

Online data submission has many advantages. Parameters and reports can be applied to real-time data requirements, so that the busy CRA can easily see what is outstanding and most pressing. Edit checks can be applied to the data as the forms are completed, with real-time feedback display to the user to request corrections. Data are received by the statistical center immediately, rather than requiring manual data entry. Form versioning can be better controlled by only displaying the version of the form that is available for submission.

SWOG uses home-grown web-based applications to register (enroll) patients, collect data, and track specimens. Each of these is discussed further below.

7.4.1 Registration

Registration of patients onto a study is the first step in data submission. Key to this process is consideration of patient eligibility. At the time of registration, the CRA will affirm that all eligibility criteria have been verified. It was once a requirement for SWOG studies to verify each individual eligibility criterion as part of the registration process, including references to specific values and dates when applicable. Despite this degree of specificity, patients were still found to be ineligible when later evaluated by the statistical center. SWOG piloted the idea of a single eligibility affirmation question and found that ineligibility rates did not increase. So, the time-consuming requirement of answering individual questions was abandoned for most studies. This practice may be necessary where more rigid reporting requirements apply, such as for FDA registration trials.

A standard set of demographics are collected at registration for all patients. These include first and last initial, race, birth date, sex, method of payment, and zip code. Full patient name and social security number are optional. Other information collected at the time of registration includes answers to stratification questions, specimen consent questions, and any additional study-specific questions required prior to enrollment. All of the information necessary to complete a registration appears on a Registration Worksheet that is included in the protocol. Clinical research associates fill out the worksheet before registering a patient so that they will be prepared for the information requested during the registration process.

The Group registration policies mentioned above are enforced at the time of registration; no exceptions are allowed. We have found that if any exceptions are ever made, we wind up arguing endlessly about what should and shouldn't be exceptions. Better to mishandle the rare case that should have been an exception than waste vast amounts of time trying to avoid mishandling the rest.

After the registration is complete, it is helpful to provide a confirmation of registration to the institution. This confirmation reiterates the treatment assignment and reminds the clinical research associate which initial materials are due and when. Immediate confirmations should result in no forgotten patients, better compliance with data submission, and quick correction if the wrong treatment arm was given mistakenly.

7.4.2 Case Report Forms

Within its EDC system, SWOG uses a "drill-down" approach to navigate to the CRFs for a study. From the data submission page, the user will first look up one or more patients to work from based on a set of parameters. These parameters include the ability to limit the patient list to those who have outstanding data expectations, or queries, which helps the CRA prioritize their work.

Once a patient is selected from that list, the application will only display the CRFs that apply. Because the patient is known at the time a CRF is selected, important header information can be prefilled for the user, saving time and guaranteeing accuracy of the data. When SWOG was receiving all patient data on paper, approximately 10% of the CRFs were received with the incorrect patient identification number, which caused delays in processing. A drill-down approach to online form selection allows these data to be completed automatically, minimizing this kind of error.

SWOG CRF design for an online setting follows a paper-based format and design. Clinical research associates appreciate the familiar layout, and while it is not encouraged, some CRAs find that it saves them time to complete the form on paper before entering the data online. When the online format matches the paper format, entry is easier and less error-prone. One consideration when designing CRFs for an online setting is whether to use a drop-down box or a set of radio buttons for a list of possible responses to a question. When selecting an option from a drop-down list, the user can inadvertently change their selection by using their mouse scroll button to move down the page. It is for this reason that SWOG forms only use radio buttons for short lists. Radio buttons also allow for the options NOT selected to appear on a printout of the page. For those CRAs compelled to keep paper records of what was submitted online, this is appreciated.

In an online environment, the CRA is not able to make comments anywhere on the page to qualify or explain any answers (or items left blank). Therefore, it is important to include a general comments section on each form for this kind of explanation, which can be important when evaluating the data.

Edit checks used on SWOG online forms come in two varieties: warnings and errors. Errors require a correction by the user, but warnings may be acknowledged by the user and the form submitted without data corrections. Because an error prevents submission of the entire form, these are applied conservatively. An error check might be used to prevent a treatment start date from being after a treatment end date, but a warning would be used to point out a deviation from the expected treatment dose. Warnings are also used instead of errors to call out values that would render the patient ineligible. It is important that the form be submittable with unexpected or outlier data so that these cases can be reported.

7.4.3 Specimens

An increasing number of SWOG studies require the collection, transfer, and analysis of various kinds of biological specimens. Therefore, SWOG has developed an interactive online application called the Specimen Tracking System to assist with the tracking of specimens. The Specimen Tracking System is used by those who submit specimens from the institutions treating patients on SWOG studies, as well as the labs and repositories that receive those specimens. The application allows specimens to be logged and indicated as shipped from any institution participating on a SWOG-coordinated study, even if the institution is not a SWOG member. Labs and repositories receiving those specimens use the application to indicate their receipt, and also to indicate if those specimens have been aliquotted and/or shipped to other labs. For studies that have eligibility, stratification, or treatment decisions dependent on assay results from specimen data, the Specimen Tracking System also collects those results and communicates instruction to the appropriate personnel.

7.4.4 Data Submission Enforcement

SWOG encourages timely submission of forms and materials from the institutions through an Expectation report. This report is available online and includes details about forms and follow-up that are due soon and that are overdue. In general, we expect baseline documentation to be submitted within 7 days. Treatment and adverse event forms generally must be submitted every 3 months while the patient is on treatment, and follow-up forms every

6 months after off treatment. Notices of events (discontinuation of treatment, recurrence, second primary, death) are due within 2 or 4 weeks of the event. The length of time a patient is followed is dependent upon the protocol; follow-up is discontinued when enough data are collected to meet the objectives for the study. Long-term survivors are followed yearly.

The Group has policies that cover institutions out of compliance with forms submission. For a given institution, if more than 10% of the patients have the baseline forms set overdue by more than 30 days, or if more than 15% of the patients on protocol treatment have follow-up overdue by more than 6 months, or if more than 20% of the patients off protocol treatment have follow-up overdue by more than 14 months, the institution is given 3 months to get caught up. If the deadline is not met, registration privileges are suspended until the institution is caught up. The threat of suspension has been a good deterrent, so hasn't often been necessary—but has been effective when imposed.

7.5 Data Evaluation

Evaluation of the patient data is probably the most important aspect of study management. Because SWOG receives its data electronically, the same research record that the data coordinator reviews is available online for the respective study coordinator to review as well. The study coordinators use an online application to review the patient records, and complete evaluation forms as necessary. Study coordinators receive monthly emails with lists of patients that require evaluation, and data coordinators receive monthly emails with lists of patients whose study coordinator evaluations have been completed. Study coordinator comments on the evaluation forms do not directly affect the database, but are reviewed by data coordinators who can make the change if they agree, or take it back to the study coordinator for discussion if they do not. Usually the data coordinators and study coordinators reach agreement on the evaluations. For the rare cases where they don't, the case can be escalated to the disease committee chair, executive officer, or even the Group chair to decide what is correct.

At the initial evaluation eligibility, stratification factors and the initial treatment dose are checked against the baseline forms. Patient events trigger further evaluations, where treatment and outcome information is abstracted. Clarification is often requested concerning missing information, causes of adverse reactions, and reasons for noncompliance. Study coordinators and data coordinators both look out for excess toxicity and misinterpretations of protocol. If problems are identified, the study coordinator submits any necessary changes or clarifications to the protocol to the operations office for distribution to the institutions.

We think this double review process works quite well. Review by data coordinators at the statistical center is important for consistency across studies within disease sites and for keeping study evaluations up to date. However, the data coordinators do not have medical expertise, so it is also important to have the study coordinator review the data. Clinical judgment is required for many aspects of evaluation, such as for serious adverse event reporting, for interpretation of pathology reports, for making judgments about circumstances not covered in response and adverse event definitions, in monitoring for excess toxicity and in recognition of clinical patterns of toxicity or response. For studies with nonstandard endpoints (such as imaging studies or secondary noncancer endpoints) additional endpoint reviews by an expert panel may also be important.

We generate a variety of reports to help in the evaluation process. Lists of which patients are due for evaluation are generated periodically. Typical times for evaluation include when the patient goes off treatment, when the patient progresses, and when the patient dies. Patient information on phase II studies is evaluated more often because of the need for closer monitoring. Other types of reports include data consistency checks that are generated periodically by study. An example of what is included in these reports might be a list of patients who went off study due to progression of disease, but do not have progression dates. Reports of possible serious adverse events that have not yet been reported to NCI are also generated for review by the operations office and study coordinator to determine if action is necessary and if so, the institution is notified.

In addition to reports, standard data summary tables are generated at least every 6 months. The tables are used both for the semiannual report of studies produced for each Group meeting and for study monitoring. Note it is possible to have standard summary tables only because we have a standard data set. Without standards the study monitoring process would be vastly more time consuming, requiring extensive programming efforts to create customized summaries for every study.

Some of the standard tables from SWOG S8811 are included in Tables 7.2–7.4. The registration, eligibility, and evaluability table (Table 7.2) reports on the number of patients registered, those found to be ineligible, and those whose data can be evaluated for various endpoints. On SWOG S8811 there was one

TABLE 7.2

Study S8811 Registration, Eligibility, and Evaluability

	Total	No Prior Chemo	Prior Chemo
Number registered	58	21	37
Ineligible	1	0	1
Eligible	57	21	36
Baseline disease assessment			
Measurable	57	21	36
Response assessment			
Adequate	44	16	28
Inadequate	13	5	8
Toxicity assessment			
Evaluable	57	21	36
Not evaluable	0	0	0

TABLE 7.3

Study S8811 Number of Patients with a Given Type and Degree of Toxicity $N = 57$

Toxicity	Grade Unknown	0	1	2	3	4	5
Abdominal pain	0	56	0	0	1	0	0
Allergy/rash	1	51	4	1	0	0	0
Alopecia	1	50	5	1	0	0	0
Anemia	0	46	3	4	3	1	0
Chills/fever	0	53	0	3	1	0	0
Diarrhea	0	21	14	15	6	1	0
Dizziness/hot flash	0	55	2	0	0	0	0
DVT	0	56	0	0	1	0	0
Granulocytopenia	0	21	6	7	9	14	0
Headache	0	56	1	0	0	0	0
Ileus/constipation	0	54	0	2	0	1	0
Lymphopenia	0	53	1	1	1	1	0
Mucositis/stomatitis	0	16	13	12	13	3	0
Nausea/vomiting	1	20	24	6	6	0	0
Thrombocytopenia	0	51	4	1	1	0	0
Weight loss	0	55	1	1	0	0	0
MAXIMUM GRADE ANY TOXICITY	1	3	9	8	20	16	0

ineligible patient (no metastatic or locally recurrent disease). Since measurable disease was required, the baseline disease status in the table is measurable for all eligible patients. The table indicates that all patients were evaluated for adverse events, but assessment for response was not as good—13 patients had disease assessments that were inadequate for the determination of response. This includes the types of patients mentioned previously—ones with unconfirmed responses, no assessments, and ones who died of other causes before response was determined.

The adverse event table (Table 7.3) gives the maximum grade of specific adverse events (there are several hundred of these, most of which won't occur

TABLE 7.4

Study S8811 Response

	No Prior Chemo	%	Prior Chemo	%
Complete response	1	5%	4	11%
Partial response	1	5%	3	8%
Unconfirmed response	1	5%	3	8%
Stable	7	33%	12	33%
Assessment inadequate	4	19%	4	11%
Increasing disease	7	33%	9	25%
Early death	0	9%	1	3%
Total	21		36	

on a specific protocol) experienced by patients on treatment. On SWOG S8811 the most commonly experienced adverse events were leukopenia, granulocytopenia, thrombocytopenia, diarrhea, mucositis, nausea, and vomiting as expected.

Response tables and survival curves are not routinely presented in the report of studies until the study is complete (per our data monitoring policy discussed in Chapter 3), but are generated for interim review by the monitoring committee (Phase II studies are monitored by a less formal committee consisting of the study coordinator, study statistician, and disease committee chair). The SWOG S8811 response table (Table 7.4) indicates there was one complete response and one partial response in the group with prior treatment for metastatic disease, and four complete responses in the no prior treatment group. The table also indicates there were four patients on the study with unconfirmed responses, eight more with inadequate disease assessment without suggestion of response, and one patient who died early. Median survival and progression-free survival on this study were 16 months and 6 months respectively (not shown).

Other tables not shown here are a patient characteristic table, which includes characteristics collected on all patients (sex, age, race, ethnicity) plus the study specific factors identified in the protocol (prior treatment groups in this case), a treatment summary table, which indicates how many patients are off treatment (all off for this study), reasons off treatment (5 due to receiving maximum planned treatment, 37 due to progression, 2 due to death, 4 due to toxicity, 9 for other reasons), and number of major deviations (none).

7.6 Publication

The final step in management and evaluation of a study is publication of the results. This involves a final clean-up of the data to resolve any outstanding evaluation questions and to bring everything up to date. It is noteworthy to mention that SWOG does not "lock" its database to new data as part of the final analysis. A snapshot of the data is captured in a SAS file and archived as a reference for that analysis. The main database is always able to accept new and updated data for a study.

The primary study analysis is dictated by the objectives and the design of the study. After the statistician analyzes the study, the study coordinator drafts a manuscript. When both the study coordinator and statistician (who are first and second authors on the paper) are satisfied with a draft, it is circulated to other authors for review and approval.

After final publication of the results of the study, and all study patients are off protocol treatment, the study status can be closed to follow-up. This removes the study from the expectation report, and any outstanding query reports, and helps clinical research associates to prioritize their efforts on more current trials.

7.7 Quality Assurance Audits

A statistical center can ensure only that the database is internally consistent. Without copies of the primary patient records, we can't be sure that what we receive matches what happens at the clinics. External audits done by clinicians are necessary to ensure this aspect of quality. Our Group recommends institutions be audited at least every three years (more often if problems are discovered). Charts reviewed should include a representative sample of patients entered on study by the institution, plus any specific charts identified by the statistical center or study coordinators as problem cases. How many charts are reviewed is, unfortunately, more a function of how much money is available than how many should be reviewed, but do note that a review of less than 10% won't be credible. In addition to chart review, compliance with regulatory requirements (e.g., drug logs) needs to be reviewed.

Review isn't sufficient of course. Standards must be established and corrective measures applied when institutions are out of compliance. Measures might include scheduling another audit in 6 months, recommendations for new procedures, or suspension of registration privileges until improvement is documented.

Detection of fraud requires extreme measures: expulsion of all involved, audit of all records from the institution, omission of all falsified data from analysis. Someone careful who is determined to falsify data is extremely difficult to detect, however. Even if auditors were to assume dishonesty, there would be time for only a superficial search for duplicate records. It is unlikely anything would be found, and the ill will generated by the assumption would be highly counterproductive to a cooperative effort. Fraud is more likely to be detected within the institution by someone whose job could be in jeopardy, so it is reasonable to establish procedures for anonymous reporting of suspected fraud. Not to minimize the seriousness of the offense—fraud is intolerable— but at least in a setting of multiple institutions and investigators the effects on a study of falsified information from a single source are diluted and should result in relatively small biases.

7.8 Training

Another important aspect of data management and quality control is training. Standardization of definitions and procedures allow development of standard training courses as well. In SWOG, training courses are presented to all new data coordinators, statisticians, clinical research associates, and study coordinators.

Data coordinator and statistician training occurs at the statistical center. The courses cover such things as the goals and history of the Group, computer training, explanations of SWOG structures and procedures, and a detailed review of SWOG standards.

Training materials are available online for institutional clinical research associates and study coordinators. Topics covered for clinical research associates include how to fill out the forms, methods for tracking down patients who are lost to follow-up, adverse event reporting, elements of informed consent, how to register patients, and how to order investigational drugs. Study coordinators are told in detail what their responsibilities will be and what policies they are expected to comply with; they are also initiated into the mysteries of protocol development and response assessment.

Training courses are a good introduction but can't possibly cover everything—thus, we maintain extensive documentation detailing responsibilities, procedures, standards, etc. for data coordinators, clinical research associates and study coordinators. We also clearly publicize our technical support email address within all of our applications. A group of statistical center staff monitors these emails and responds to them within 24 hours of receipt. Some of the best ideas for enhancements to our applications come from the users.

7.9 Database Management

The field of database management is a highly specialized one with a large literature and a language all its own. We will only touch on some of the more important aspects, focusing on computerized database management for organizations carrying out multiple clinical trials, whether in single institutions or in cooperative groups. A good review of this field is given by McFadden et al., 1995.

7.9.1 Database Structures

The software used by most trial organizations today is one of several commercially available relational database management systems. The relational model can be thought of simply as organizing data into tables that can be linked to other tables by certain key variables. For example, the SWOG database has a table for data unique to a patient (patient identifier, sex, age, race, vital status, last contact date, etc.) and other tables for data unique to a patient on a given study, such as the adverse event table (patient identifier, study number, types and degrees of adverse events) and the evaluation table (patient identifier, study number, eligibility, time to progression, etc.). Data from the patient table can be linked to these other tables through the patient identifier. This kind of structure is highly flexible (tables can be added as needed) and very intuitive; there is a close correspondence between many of the tables and the data collection forms. Retrieval of data for analysis is a matter of specifying and linking the relevant tables. The relational model is thus particularly suited to statistical analysis, as opposed to hierarchical databases. Hierarchical structure consists of a pyramid of record types, where each record type is "owned" by the record type next up in the hierarchy. For instance if the basic unit (highest record type) is the patient, the first record type might be characteristics of the patient that do not change (sex, date and type of diagnosis, etc.), the next might be visit basics (date of visit, BSA, etc.), the next level outcomes from the visit (lab values, agents and doses administered, etc.). Hierarchical databases that are patient-oriented are more suited to retrieving data on individual patients (e.g., for clinical use) than for retrieving data for analysis. For instance, accessing a single adverse event table for analysis is much more straightforward than identifying all visits for which patients were on a particular study and summarizing adverse events from those visits. A hierarchical structure with study as the basic unit is better but not ideal when patients can be on multiple studies, because information that does not change for a patient must be repeated for each study. This kind of structure is also not ideal when the same forms are used for multiple studies as the same table cannot be used for all occurrences of the same form. For more information about the advantages of the relational model for clinical trials organizations see Blumenstein (1989).

The concept of referential integrity is an important one in a relational database structure. If patient-specific data (sex, birth date, etc.) resides in one table, and adverse events pertaining to those patients reside in another table, there will be a link between the two, such as a numeric patient identifier. Relational databases will allow a constraint to be placed on the adverse event table that disallows any records with patient identifiers that do not first exist in the patient table. This kind of constraint is called a foreign key, and is important to use wisely in a relational database structure so as to prevent the entry of incorrect data. In this case, such a constraint would prevent adverse event records for nonexistent patients, an important rule to enforce.

As mentioned previously, SWOG receives most of its patient data through an online interface. This includes the ability to receive submissions that result in error or warning messages, and display the erroneous data back to the user for correction. This kind of feature requires that we save the data from the unsuccessful submission attempts. We use a mirror set of "staging tables" to collect all the submissions from the application. If all edit checks are passed, the data are promoted to the "active tables" from which data coordinators, statisticians, and study coordinators do their work. This distinction is important so that data that are successfully submitted do not mingle with data that failed submission checks.

7.10 Conclusion

It bears repeating that the protocol document sets the standard for the conduct of the clinical trial. A clear and concise protocol that has been reviewed and agreed upon by the entire study team will get any clinical trial off on the right track. Protocol amendments are often required, but the more rigorous review can be prior to the first enrollment, the better.

No protocol document is complete without a set of case report forms that will be used to submit the study data. Case report forms should get the same level of review as the protocol document itself, and reflect standard formatting and terminology. Only the data items relevant to the conduct of the study need be collected. "Extra" data items only serve to spread the clinical research associate's attention too thin, and threaten the accuracy of the data which actually impact the analysis. The method of submission should be clear in the protocol and well supported by necessary documentation and training.

Once received at the central statistical center, data should undergo further review by trained professional staff to code standard summary variables, search for inconsistencies, and query for necessary corrections or clarifications. This level of review imposes consistency within the study and across other studies, and complements a medical review of the data. Medical review should be done to review dosing, adverse events, and other aspects of patient care, followed by changes to the protocol as necessary. Neither of these reviews compares the research record to the clinical record, and periodic audits against a representative sample of cases at the participating institutions should be conducted.

With a solid protocol document, well-designed case report forms, an appropriate reliable database, and a well-trained study team, the clinical trial will yield a reliable result, and be suitable for publication and furtherance of knowledge in the fight against cancer.

8

Reporting of Results

Cave quid dicis, quando, et cui.

The reporting of the results from a clinical trial is one of the most anxiously awaited aspects of the clinical trials process. This reporting can take on many forms: reports to investigators during the conduct of the trial; interim outcome reports to the Data Monitoring Committee; abstracts submitted to scientific meetings; and finally, the published report in the medical literature. For any type of study report, it is important to recognize what type of information is appropriate to transmit, and how that information can be communicated in the most scientifically appropriate fashion. In 2001 an international committee comprised of clinical trialists, statisticians, epidemiologists, and editors of biomedical journals reviewed the quality of reporting for randomized clinical trials. The result of this review led to two publications under the title of CONSORT (Consolidated Standards for Reporting Trials). The CONSORT statement proposes a flow diagram for reporting trials, and a checklist of necessary items. The checklist and explanatory article have been updated since 2001 (Schulz et al., 2010; Moher et al., 2010) to improve clarity and incorporate recommendations on new topics (see also Simon and Wittes, 1985).

For routine reports, accrual, ineligibility, major protocol deviations, and toxicity should be presented. Such reports are important for early identification of excess toxicity, ambiguities in the protocol, and other study management problems; this is discussed in Chapter 7. In this chapter, we concentrate on interim (to the Data Monitoring Committee) and final reports on the major trial endpoints. Information in these reports should allow the reader to evaluate the trial: its design, conduct, data collection, analysis, and interpretation. While there are no absolute standards for the reporting of clinical trials, there are some basics regarding timing and content that should be observed.

8.1 Timing of Report

Once a trial has been opened, researchers turn their attention to the design of future trials, and are impatient for any clues that the current trial can provide for new study design. Thus, almost from the beginning of patient accrual, there is pressure to report any data accumulated so far. As discussed in Chapter 6, a common problem in Phase III reporting has stemmed from a tendency to report primary outcome results while a trial is still accruing patients, or after study closure but before the data have "matured." Accrual may be affected and too many incorrect conclusions may be drawn when results are reported early. The use of monitoring committees and appropriate stopping rules minimizes such problems.

Early reporting causes similar problems in Phase II studies. Consider a trial designed to accrue 40 patients with advanced colorectal cancer. Of the first 25 patients accrued, 15 have gone off study and are evaluable for response, while the other 10 are either still on treatment, or have not had their records updated sufficiently to assess response. These 10 patients are not necessarily the last 10 to have registered—they might include patients who have been on therapy for a long time, patients who have poor compliance regarding return visits, or patients for whom required tests have been run, but have not yet been reported. Moreover, there may be a tendency for institutions to report the negative results first (less documentation is required). If this is the case, then the response proportion in the first 15 patients may be pessimistic as an estimate of the true response probability. The early pessimism may even result in changes in the types of patient registered to the study. For example, patients with less severe disease may now be put on trials perceived to be more promising. This change in patient population could lead to the registration of patients who are less likely to respond, resulting in a final response estimate that remains overly pessimistic. Thus, as for Phase III studies, care should be taken not to report results until the data are mature.

The definition of mature data is dependent upon the type of study being conducted, and should be specified prior to the opening of the trial. No matter the definition, however, the principle to be strictly enforced is that outcome information should not be reported until the study is closed to accrual, and the appropriate reporting time has been reached. This rule limits biases in the final outcome of the trial that can occur when early data are released.

8.1.1 Phase II Trials

Typical Phase II trials have either response, progression-free survival or survival as the endpoint. For two-stage designs (commonly used for studies of investigational new drugs), reporting only occurs once permanent closure has taken place, and all registered patients have been evaluated. Outcomes are never reported at the conclusion of the first stage of accrual (unless the study closes after the first stage), for the reasons given above. Specific rules, which are established during the study planning phase, specify the results needed to continue to the second stage of accrual. When it is determined that accrual should continue, the actual number of observed responses or events is not reported; investigators are only informed that the minimum number of responses necessary for continuation has been observed and that the study will continue to completion. Once the study has closed and all patients have been evaluated for response, the final study report is prepared for presentation at professional meetings and for publication in the medical literature.

8.1.2 Phase III Trials

Phase III trials typically last for many years, making the desire for early reporting even more acute. The literature is replete with examples of studies that reported early promising results, only to have those results negated once additional follow-up was available. SWOG S7924 (a study of radiotherapy versus no radiotherapy after complete response to chemotherapy in patients with limited small-cell lung cancer) is an example. This was reported in ASCO abstracts as promising during accrual to the study (Kies et al., 1982) and positive after accrual (Mira et al., 1984). The conclusion after the final analysis, however, was that there was no survival benefit due to radiotherapy (Kies et al., 1987). (SWOG no longer allows reports of study outcomes until accrual has been completed and the study has reached maturity.) The timing of study reports should be defined in the study protocol, including the time of final analysis and times of interim analyses. At interim analysis times confidential outcome analyses are provided to the study's Data Monitoring Committee (see Chapter 6). Only if this committee recommends early reporting (based on predefined guidelines) may the results of the study be released prior to the final analysis time defined in the protocol.

8.2 Required Information

The amount of detail in a report will vary according to its purpose. In general, though, it will be important to include the following information.

8.2.1 Objectives and Design

The aims of the trial should be stated in any report or manuscript (in both abstract and methods sections for a manuscript). Primary and secondary endpoints should be clearly defined. Response and toxicity in particular require definition, as so many variations of these are in use. If explanation is necessary, the relation of the endpoints to the objectives of the study should be stated.

The study design should be described, including whether the study is a Phase II or Phase III trial and if there are any predefined patient subsets with separate accrual goals. The target sample size should be given (for each subset if applicable), along with justification (precision of estimation, or level of test and power for a specified alternative). The interim analysis plan, if any, should be specified. For Phase III trials, some details of the randomization scheme should be given, including whether or not the randomization was balanced on stratification factors, and how that balance was achieved (see Chapter 3 for a discussion of randomization schemes).

Decision rules and trial characteristics for multi-arm studies should be described, and if a strategy for testing multiple endpoints was specified in the protocol, this should also be included.

8.2.2 Eligibility and Treatment

A definition of the patient population under study is provided by a clear description of the eligibility criteria. Among the items that should be included are the site, histology, and stage of disease under study, any prior therapy restrictions, baseline laboratory values required for patient eligibility, and medical conditions contraindicating patient participation on the trial.

The details of the treatments should also be defined (not just "5-FU therapy"), including dose, schedule, method of delivery, and required supportive therapy (e.g., hydration, growth factors). In the final manuscript, dose modification plans should also be included.

8.2.3 Results

The results section should include the timing of the report, i.e., whether it is the planned final analysis, a planned interim analysis to the DMC, or, if neither of these, the justification for the early report. The results section should also include the time interval over which patients were accrued, the total number of patients registered in that period, the numbers of patients ineligible and reasons for ineligibility. If any eligible patients are excluded from analyses the reasons for the exclusions should be given (there should be very few of these; see below for guidelines).

Since eligibility criteria allow for a variety of patients to be entered on trial, a summary of basic characteristics of patients actually accrued is necessary to indicate the risk status of the final sample. Examples of variables to include are patient demographics (age, sex, race, ethnicity), stratification factors, and other important descriptive factors (e.g., performance status, extent of disease, number of prior treatment regimens). For randomized trials, a statement on how well balanced the treatment arms are with respect to basic characteristics should also be included. However, we do not recommend testing the balance and using an adjusted test if significant. If this approach to testing is not prespecified, testing with and without adjustment may inflate the significance level. If it is prespecified so only one test is done, it doesn't help much—the effect on power is generally small (Permutt, 1990). A significant imbalance either means the randomization was improperly done (in which case adjusting won't fix the problem) or that the imbalance is a random event, which is expected to happen on occasion in randomized trials; it does not mean adjustment is necessary. Consider also that lack of significance does not mean adjustment is unnecessary; highly prognostic variables may impact results regardless of balance.

The text should also contain a summary of the treatment experience. This summary should include a report on the number of patients who completed therapy as planned, and the numbers and reasons for early termination of therapy. Reasons for early termination might include toxicity, death not due to disease, or patient refusal. For Phase III trials, if large numbers of patients have failed to complete therapy, some comparison between treatment arms with respect to patient compliance may be of interest. However, comparisons of treatment within compliance subsets should not be presented (see Chapter 9 for an explanation of this pitfall). A summary of deviations to protocol specifications should also be included. Definitions of "protocol deviation" may vary, and are rather subjective. Thus, a definition of what constitutes a deviation is appropriate in this summary.

The number of patients evaluated for toxicity, the number with adequate response and progression/relapse information and an indication of maturity of follow-up should be provided. This last typically would include the number dead and the number lost to follow-up, plus minimum, maximum and median follow-up time. However, there is some debate on how to calculate median follow-up time (Schemper and Smith, 1996.) Among the ways to estimate this is to compute the median follow-up only for patients who remain alive (which we prefer), or compute the median of time from registration to last contact date (without regard to survival status). The manuscript should specify what statistic is being used. Some or all of survival, progression-free survival, response and toxicity are generally primary and secondary outcomes in a trial; these should be summarized as discussed in the analysis section below. Exploratory results should be relegated to a separate section of the results and be accompanied by numerous statements minimizing the importance of anything observed.

8.3 Analyses

8.3.1 Exclusions, Intent to Treat

All patients entered onto the trial should be accounted for. In general, all eligible patients are included in any analyses from a study. This is the well-established intent-to-treat principle, which is the only method of analysis that eliminates selection bias. An alternate definition of intent-to-treat proposes including all randomized patients regardless of eligibility. We find it unconvincing to include a patient who may have the wrong disease, stage or other relevant, protocol specified disease characteristics. There may be some legitimate reasons for patient exclusions for other than eligibility in certain analyses, however. For example, when estimating toxicity probabilities, it usually makes sense to exclude patients who were never treated. Keep in mind, though, that patient exclusions often can contribute to biased estimates of outcomes.

For Phase II trials with the goal of evaluating drug activity, all eligible patients who receive drug should be included in the analyses. A bias in response probability estimates is caused when patients for whom response was not evaluable are excluded. Since the reasons for not being evaluable generally are indicative of treatment failure (death prior to formal tests of disease assessment, early progression, or early refusal of treatment), the result of excluding these patients from the analysis is that the response estimates are inflated. An American Society of Clinical Oncology abstract in the treatment of hepatocellular carcinoma with a thymidylate synthetase inhibitor reported responses in 8% of 13 evaluable patients (Stuart et al., 1996). However, this study had enrolled 24 patients, 8 of whom had been judged to be inevaluable due to toxicity or rapid disease progression and 3 of whom were too early for evaluation. If one assumes that all 8 of the patients with toxicity or rapid progression failed to respond to therapy, then a revised response estimate becomes $1/21 = 5\%$, over a third less than the original estimate. Why is the original estimate in error? The goal of Phase II studies is to decide whether to continue study of the regimen. The decision is based on whether sufficient activity is observed in the type of patient defined by the eligibility criteria. The goal is not to estimate the response probability in the subgroup of patients who, after the fact, are known not to progress too fast on therapy, and not to develop early toxicities. (If this were the goal, then eligibility would have to include a requirement that patients be succeeding on the regimen for a specified time before registration is allowed.) The after-the-fact response probability might hold some interest, but it is useless for deciding whether a new patient should be treated with the regimen. We want the estimate that most nearly matches the prediction we can make for an individual patient prior to receiving drug, not the estimate we can give of what the chances are of response if they don't fail right away.

For Phase III trials, which by definition are comparative, the intent-to-treat principle states that all eligible patients are analyzed according to the arm to which they are randomized, even if the patient refuses therapy according to that arm, or even if their treatment involves a major deviation from protocol specifications. It is important to stress that eligibility is based on patient characteristics or tests done prior to registration. For example, a pathology specimen obtained prior to registration, but read as ineligible by the pathologist after a patient has been registered still means the patient is not eligible. The determination of ineligibility relates to the timing of patient information, not the timing of the review.

The reason behind the intent-to-treat concept is to avoid the bias that can occur by arm-specific selective deviations or refusals. Reasons for treatment deviations cannot be assumed to be random. High risk patients might be more likely than low risk patients to refuse assignment to a less aggressive treatment arm, for instance, or very good risk patients might decide toxicity is not worth whatever small benefit from treatment they might expect. Patient groups defined by initial treatment assignment are approximately comparable with respect to pretreatment characteristics because of the randomization; systematically throwing some patients out of the study destroys that comparability. Note intent-to-treat does NOT mean that ineligible patients must be included in the analysis. It means that treatment received AFTER randomization (or anything else that happens after randomization for that matter) cannot be used as a reason to exclude patients. No systematic bias should occur when patients on all treatment arms are omitted based on events or characteristics that occur or are collected prior to registration—randomization takes care of that. Although analyses using all randomized patients may be required, it may be detrimental to leave ineligible patients in the primary analyses—it becomes impossible to characterize what type of patient the sample represents, and might mask whatever treatment effect there is.

8.3.2 Summary Statistics: Estimates and Variability of Estimates

For Phase II trials, the primary outcome measure is usually response, or progression-free or overall survival. When it is response, the report should include the estimate of the response probability (number of responses/number of eligible patients), as well as progression-free and overall survival curves if these are specified as important secondary endpoints. Survival should be included if response is the primary endpoint, since survival is usually an important secondary endpoint. For Phase III trials, all major endpoints should be presented by treatment arm, along with estimates of medians and/or hazard ratio estimates for time-to-event endpoints. Estimates of differences adjusted for important prognostic factors are also often appropriate. When the proportional hazards model is correct, adjusting for important prognostic factors in a Cox model provides a better estimate of treatment effect (Anderson et al., 2006).

There is often a temptation to provide survival curves for responders versus nonresponders. However, as discussed in Chapter 9, such comparisons are virtually meaningless. Duration of response out of context with the rest of the times to failure aren't particularly useful either. Instead, a progression-free survival curve based on all patients on trial should be given. The "durable responses" will appear on these curves as late failures. The duration-of-response information is still there, while the additional failures provide information on what proportion of patients are early and late failures—thus you get a more complete picture of the results of the trial than an estimate based only on responders.

For both Phase II and Phase III studies toxicity summary information is important. More detailed summaries generally are required for Phase II studies, for which further characterization of toxicity of the regimen typically is a goal. An exhaustive list of toxicities observed on the study, including all degrees of toxicity, may be in order. For Phase III studies employing only well-characterized treatment agents, it may be sufficient to report the number of patients with high degrees of common toxicities, plus any unexpected toxicities of any degree that were observed.

For quality of life (QOL) endpoints, a description of the QOL instrument and its properties (reliability, validity, and sensitivity to change in patient status) should be provided, as should the timing of assessments and compliance with filling out the forms. Summary of QOL data is particularly challenging due to the fact that these data are often missing and that this missingness is not random, but related to the endpoint. Patients may not fill out forms due to factors related to poor quality of life (such as deterioration due to disease, excess toxicity, depression or death) or due to factors related to good quality of life (such as going on vacation when the form is due).

In analyzing change in QOL from baseline to subsequent times, estimates are biased if either all patients at baseline are compared to all patients who fill out forms at each time, or if only patients with both baseline and all subsequent forms are used in the comparison. In the first case, if patients with seriously decreased quality of life at time T do not fill out forms, the average at time T is biased toward good QOL and any favorable difference between baseline and time T is an overestimate. In the second, differences between baseline and time T in the subset of patients who filled out all forms may not reflect differences in the whole group; in this case it may be less clear which way the bias goes, but typically this also overestimates any improvement.

An approach to examining QOL data that addresses some of the difficulties and allows for identification of bias involves summarizing according to the drop-out pattern and reason for drop-out. Averages for patients with only baseline and the first assessment are presented, along with averages for patients with only baseline plus the first and second assessments, and so on, which constitute a more comprehensive summary of the results than the simpler approaches often used. The averages can be restricted further according to reasons for drop-out. Such summaries often reveal worse QOL for early drop-outs, decreased QOL at the time of last completed assessment, and steeper decline when the reason for discontinuing QOL assessments is due to illness or death. All of these indicate drop-out is related to QOL. Figure 8.1, adapted from part of a figure in Moinpour et al. (2000), shows the result of such a strategy for a measure of symptom distress collected in SWOG 8905

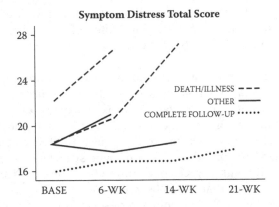

FIGURE 8.1
Example of biased follow-up due to nonrandomly missing QOL data.

(Leichman et al., 1995), a study of 5-FU in advanced colon cancer. The two dashed lines give the symptom distress score for patients who discontinued follow-up due to death or illness, with separate plots for patients who completed two or three QOL questionnaires. These two lines show higher baseline values (corresponding to worse symptom distress), and steeper slopes than the solid lines, which represent patients who dropped out after 2 or 3 visits for other reasons. Patients who completed follow-up (dotted plot) started with the lowest baseline values, and had the flattest slopes over time. Analysis methods using models that incorporate patterns of drop-out are becoming common. (See Troxel et al., 1998, and Hogan and Laird, 1997, for discussions of issues and methods.)

Perhaps the most important summary information in a report is an indication of how reliable the results are. Generally this is done with confidence intervals (see Chapter 2) for the reported estimates. An estimated treatment hazard ratio of 1.9 with a confidence interval of 0.94–3.8, for instance, could be interpreted as exciting if the confidence interval were not reported. When the confidence interval is reported it becomes clear the result is highly unreliable (consistent with no difference at all as well as with an astonishing benefit) and worth at most guarded optimism, not excitement. While it is always important to report confidence intervals, it is absolutely critical to report them to the data monitoring committee for interim reports lest early trends be over-interpreted. For these the confidence intervals should not be the standard 95% intervals, but should reflect the early conservatism built into the design. If a test of level 0.01 is being done at an interim analysis, then a 99% confidence interval is more suitable than a 95% interval.

Estimation and confidence intervals when interim analyses are part of the design brings up a difficult statistical issue. If a study continues after the first interim analysis, then one decision has already been made that results are not consistent with very small response probabilities (Phase II) or that differences are not exceptionally large (Phase III with early stopping for positive results). Incorporation of these observations into estimates at the next interim analysis time tends to increase the response estimate and shift up the confidence interval a bit (Phase II) or decrease the difference estimate and shift down the confidence interval a bit (Phase III). The statistical difficulty is that there is no unique or even standard way to do this. For example, Jennison and Turnbull (1983), Chang and O'Brien (1986), and Duffy and Santner (1987) propose three different ways to adjust confidence intervals to account for two-stage Phase II designs. The biggest differences in adjusted and unadjusted intervals generally occur when results at later analysis times become extreme (e.g., if there are no responses in the second stage of accrual in a Phase II study after several in the first stage, or if a very large difference is observed at the final analysis of a Phase III following only modest differences at earlier analyses). In some cases it might be worth adjusting, but in practice we expect that if conservative early stopping rules are used, then unadjusted intervals will present a reasonable impression of the results of the study (Green, 2006).

8.3.3 Interpretation of Results

8.3.3.1 One-Sided versus Two-Sided Tests

The choice of whether to perform a one-sided or two-sided test is determined during study development, and should be specified in the statistical considerations section of the protocol. The one-sided p-value for the test of the primary endpoint should be reported for a study designed with a one-sided hypothesis. The possible conclusions from such a study are "the experimental treatment has been shown to be better, use it" and "the experimental treatment has not been shown to be better, stick with the standard." If the experimental arm appears worse than the control, this will mean the p-value is close to 1 rather than being close to 0. The possibility that the experimental arm is actually worse may be of some interest but does not represent one of the decisions used to plan the statistical error rates for the trial. In a multi-arm setting with an ordered hypothesis, think of "one-sided" as "ordered" instead and the same comments apply. Either conclude there is evidence for the hypothesized ordering or not; changing the ordering after the fact invalidates the design considerations.

A two-sided p-value should be reported for a study designed with a two-sided hypothesis. The possible conclusions for a two-arm trial are "arm A is better, use it," "arm B is better, use it" and "there is insufficient evidence to conclude either one is better, use either." The possible conclusions from a multi-arm trial are not so simply listed. If a global test (all arms equal versus not all arms equal) is planned first, one possible conclusion is "there is insufficient evidence to conclude any of the arms are inferior or superior"; after this the possible outcomes will depend on the specific hypotheses stated in the protocol.

The primary test statistic reported for a Phase III trial should be either an unadjusted logrank test if simple randomization was used, or a stratified logrank or Cox model adjusting for the stratification factors if randomization followed a stratified scheme. Failure to adjust for variables used in the randomization results in conservative testing when the stratification factors have strong prognostic effects (Anderson et al., 2006).

For any trial, the testing strategy specified in the protocol must be followed. For instance, if a two-sided test is specified, claims based on one-sided testing cannot be made, or if a gate-keeper approach is used and the first test is not significant, then claims of significance cannot be made for the next level of testing. In addition, the test specified in the protocol must be used. For a two-arm trial this is often a logrank or stratified logrank test (see Chapter 2). When proportional hazards assumptions don't appear to be met after a study is complete, it is tempting to use a test other than the logrank test to improve power. However, using a second test, especially one based on looking at the data, means an extra opportunity for a false positive error, making the significance level specified in the design incorrect. To allow for two tests the study must be designed for two tests—with levels for each adjusted so that the overall false positive probability for the study (probability either test rejects when there are no differences) is the desired level α.

8.3.3.2 Positive, Negative, and Equivocal Trials

Positive results on a Phase II or a two-arm Phase III study are relatively easy to define. If the protocol-specified hypothesis test of the protocol-specified primary endpoint is significant using protocol-specified levels, the result is positive. The definition of negative is not so easy. What distinguishes a negative trial from an equivocal trial is the extent of the confidence interval around the null hypothesis value. On a two-arm Phase III trial the null hypothesis generally is that the death hazard ratio equals 1. Thus for a trial in which the null hypothesis of treatment equality cannot be rejected, a confidence interval for the hazard ratio that contains only values close to 1 constitutes a negative trial; if some values are not close to 1 the trial is equivocal. One should never conclude there is "no difference" between treatment arms—the confidence interval never consists precisely of the value 1. Similarly, a Phase II trial is convincingly negative if all values in the confidence interval are close to p_0 and equivocal if not.

What is "close" and what is "not close" is a matter of clinical judgment, but for a well-designed trial with high power against sensible alternatives, these can be interpreted as "less than the difference specified in the alternative hypothesis" and "greater than the difference specified in the alternative hypothesis," respectively. In this case, a confidence interval lying entirely below the alternative would constitute evidence of a negative result. If power for the alternative is high, failure to reject the null hypothesis will generally result in such confidence intervals (unless the p-value is close to α). Trials that are too small to have good power for reasonable alternatives, however, stand a good chance of being interpreted as equivocal if the null hypothesis is not rejected. For example an adjuvant trial designed to have 80% power to detect a hazard ratio of 1.5 may well turn out not to reject the null hypothesis, but the confidence interval may contain hazard ratios on the order of 1.25, a difference many would argue is clinically important. Be very careful not to overinterpret trials of inadequate size that don't reject the null hypothesis.

A multi-arm trial is positive if a superior arm is identified according to the design criteria. It is negative if the differences among arms are not consistent with a moderate benefit due to any one of the arms over another. In practice it is very hard to conclude that a multi-arm trial is anything but equivocal. Variability guarantees differences between the arms, and chances are some of these will be large enough not to exclude differences of interest unless the sample size is very large. Furthermore, even if a protocol specified test statistic is significant, readers may not be persuaded that the hypothesized best arm truly is best unless stricter testing is also significant. For instance, suppose a test of equality against an ordered alternative, A < AB < ABC, rejects in favor of the alternative. According to the design, ABC should be concluded the best arm. If, however, ABC were only a little better than AB (and not significant in a pairwise comparison), there would be doubt as to whether adding C to the regimen was necessary.

8.3.3.3 *Multiple Endpoints*

In general there should be only one primary endpoint for a trial, the one on which sample size and statistical error rates are based. However, there are usually several important secondary endpoints. Results for each endpoint should be presented separately, not combined into some arbitrary aggregate (see also Chapter 5). If analyses of all endpoints lead to the same conclusion, there is no problem of interpretation. A positive result in the primary endpoint not accompanied by positive results in secondary endpoints is still positive, but may be viewed with less enthusiasm. For instance, a new agent found to have a modest survival advantage over a standard agent but with a serious toxicity increase or a decrease in quality of life will likely be concluded useful, but less useful than if there had been no difference in toxicity or quality of life. On the other hand, if there is no significant difference in the primary endpoint, then results are still negative, but differences in secondary endpoints might be useful in making clinical decisions concerning what regimen to use.

8.3.4 Secondary Analyses

Everything but the intent-to-treat analysis of all eligible patients with respect to the protocol-specified primary endpoint using the protocol-specified test is a secondary or exploratory analysis. In addition to protocol specified secondary analyses, there are frequent requests for additional tests during the analysis phase of the trial. One of the most common such requests is to evaluate treatment results within subsets of patients (including stratification factors).

The most common mistake in the analysis of subsets is to perform a test of treatment effect separately within levels of the variable of interest. For example, if it is thought that treatment may vary by sex, the temptation is to produce (and test) a separate set of survival curves for men and women. This strategy yields tests that have poor power and inflated level (see Section 9.5). The safest strategy is to perform a test of interaction between treatment and the variable(s) of interest. A test of interaction tests whether the magnitude of the treatment effect (hazard ratio) differs between levels of the factor. A nonsignificant test of interaction suggests there is no evidence of differences in effect of treatment within subsets, and further exploration should stop. (Note the cautious wording "no evidence of differences." As for any nonsignificant test with low power, interpretation of a nonsignificant result is not equivalent to proving "no difference.")

For all but the primary endpoint, results of any exploratory analyses must be viewed and reported with caution. Although an occasional new insight is uncovered, data dredging leads to mainly incorrect conclusions (see Chapter 9). Care should be taken to report only strong statistical associations with plausible biological explanations, and even then the observations should be reported as exploratory, needing confirmation in other studies.

8.4 Conclusion

The introductory quote means "be careful what you say, when, and to whom." Treatment and management decisions will be made based on what you report. Given the long history of premature enthusiasm and exaggerated claims for new treatments in cancer, there is reason to take every care that conclusions do not go beyond what your trial data support. Patients' lives may depend on it.

9

Pitfalls

The crooks already know these tricks; honest men must learn them in self-defense.

—**Darrel Huff (1954)**

9.1 Introduction

The results of a well-designed and executed clinical trial should be evident from a couple of summary statistics—but stopping at those summaries in a manuscript is rare. It is reasonable to want to see if more can be learned from a long, expensive effort. The temptation to over-interpret secondary analyses can be irresistible. Exploring data and analyzing different endpoints does sometimes lead to new insights; instead, far too often, it leads to implausible hypotheses and faulty conclusions. In this chapter we discuss problems with some common types of analyses which have been used to try to draw treatment conclusions beyond those supported by the study design. In Chapter 10 we discuss methods for exploratory data analysis.

9.2 Historical Controls

As noted in Chapter 3, any nonrandomized choice of a control group will be systematically different from the experimental group in countless ways, some known, many unmeasurable. We know from numerous examples that there are historical trends in disease incidence and survival that are difficult to explain. For example, diphtheria is a heterogeneous disease caused by several bacteria which vary in deadliness. The bacteria were discovered in 1894 and antiserum was produced and made available in Europe in 1894–1895. Mortality due to diphtheria decreased at this time—but the decline had started *before* the introduction of antiserum. The prevalences of the various types of bacteria were changing, making the contribution of treatment uncertain. Thirty years later it was still unknown whether treatment helped, as deaths in

169

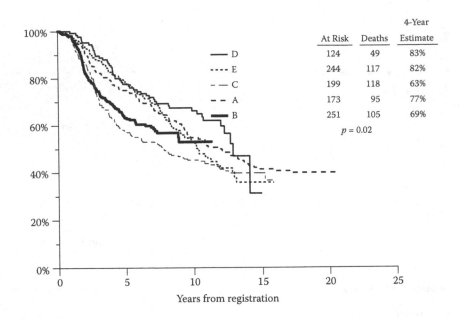

FIGURE 9.1
Survival distributions for CMFVP arms of five SWOG breast cancer trials.

1924 had risen to 1871 levels (Lancaster, 1994). While historical controls may be useful for some Phase II designs (see Chapter 5), it is rare that new treatments should be adopted without a well-defined randomized Phase III trial.

For a modern cancer example, Figure 9.1 shows the CMFVP arms from five SWOG adjuvant breast cancer studies done in node positive patients between 1975 and 1989 (Rivkin et al., 1989; Rivkin et al., 1993; Budd et al., 1995; Rivkin et al., 1994; Rivkin et al., 1996). Survival differs widely despite use of the same treatment in the same stage of disease in the same cooperative group. At the time of the first study, single agent LPAM was standard adjuvant treatment. If the worst of the CMFVP arms had been compared to historical experience on LPAM, combination chemotherapy would have been concluded to be no better (Figure 9.2); fortunately a randomized trial was done, and the appropriate comparison (arm A, Figure 9.3) demonstrated superiority of CMFVP.

Some of the reasons for the differences between the CMFVP arms are clear— studies B and C consisted of estrogen receptor-negative patients (who generally have a less favorable prognosis), D and E required estrogen receptor-positive disease, and study A was a mixture. Unfortunately, identifying the biases is not always so easy. Between 1977 and 1989 SWOG did a series of four Phase III trials with the same eligibility criteria in multiple myeloma (Salmon et al., 1983; Durie et al., 1986; Salmon et al., 1990; Salmon et al., 1994). Figure 9.4 shows survival on the four studies (arms combined). The estimates of the survival distributions of the four studies are nearly the same; it would appear that little progress was made in myeloma treatment during this time. Contrast this with Figure 9.5, which shows survival on the arm common to each

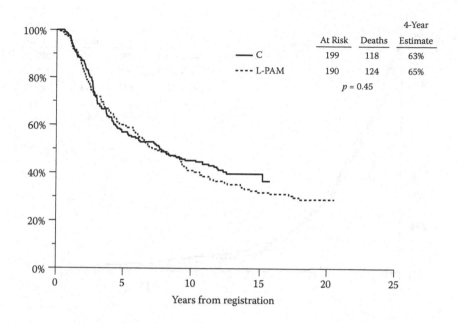

FIGURE 9.2
Survival distributions for worst arm of CMFVP versus L-PAM based on five SWOG breast cancer trials.

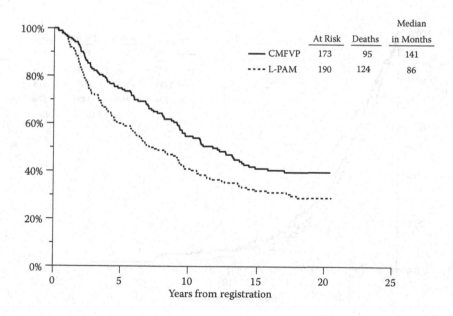

FIGURE 9.3
Survival distributions based on randomized comparison of CMFVP versus L-PAM on SWOG breast cancer trial S7436.

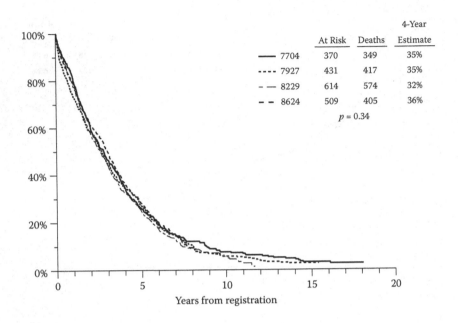

FIGURE 9.4
Survival distributions for four successive SWOG myeloma trials.

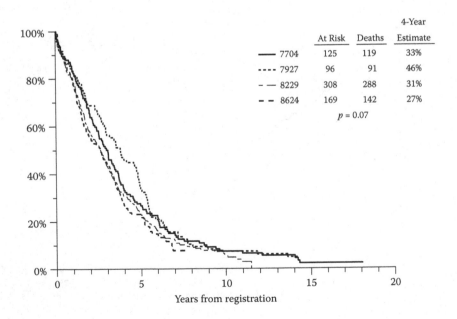

FIGURE 9.5
Survival distributions for common VMCP/VBAP arms of four successive SWOG myeloma trials.

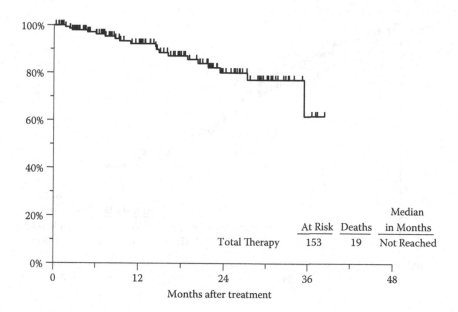

FIGURE 9.6
Survival distribution for pilot trial of high-dose therapy in myeloma.

of the trials. Despite the same eligibility, the same treatment, and largely the same participating institutions, the survival curves on the four arms appear quite different—almost statistically significant at the conventional 0.05 level! If comparability can't be counted on in this ideal setting, it certainly can't be counted on when control groups are chosen arbitrarily from the literature or from convenient databases.

The next examples illustrate the potential magnitude of selection bias in historical comparisons. Consider results in Figure 9.6 from a myeloma pilot study of high dose therapy with autologous bone marrow transplant (Barlogie et al., 1995). Viewed next to standard results in Figure 9.4, transplant results appear quite promising. Is this observation sufficient to declare transplant the new standard without doing a randomized trial of transplant versus a standard chemotherapy control group? Would it be unethical to do a randomized trial of transplant versus control? When the difference is this large it is tempting to conclude that results couldn't all be due to systematic biases. Figure 9.7 suggests otherwise, however. Major sources of bias in the historical comparison are the different eligibility criteria for the two types of trials. Potential transplant patients must be young and in good condition; criteria for standard therapy are not so strict. Figure 9.7 shows how results on one possible historical control arm (VAD, one of the arms of SWOG S8624, and the induction arm for the transplant protocol) look when restricted to patients under 70 years of age with good renal function. Results look quite a bit better for standard therapy—and this is after adjustment for just two known biases.

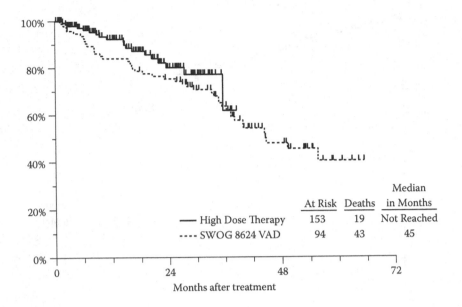

FIGURE 9.7
Survival distributions for historical comparison of high-dose therapy with standard therapy for myeloma, using only patients under 70 and with good renal function.

Unknown and unmeasurable selection factors may play an even larger role, so a randomized trial coordinated by SWOG was conducted to answer the question. Figure 9.8 shows the results from SWOG S9321 (Barlogie et al., 2006), demonstrating comparable results between high-dose therapy with melphalan and total body irradiation followed by autologous transplantation, and standard dose therapy.

Now consider the sequence of curves in Figures 9.9–9.11 from a pilot study in limited small-cell lung cancer (McCracken et al., 1990). The first figure (Figure 9.9) shows survival for all patients on the study; median survival was 18 months. Transplant advocates claimed that survival on high-dose therapy might be two to three times longer than on standard treatment. In order to get high-dose therapy plus transplant on most pilot studies, however, patients had to have been in good physical condition, and must have received and responded to induction treatment with conventional chemotherapy. Figure 9.10 shows survival on the SWOG pilot when restricted to patients with good performance status who survived four months. It is evident that these requirements select out a relatively good risk subset of patients; median survival for this subset is 26 months. (Note: We could make this look even better by including the four months the patients were being treated on induction.) Results improve even more (Figure 9.11) when patients are further restricted to those with disease in complete response at four months; we're now up to a median of 48 months, 2.7 times the median on standard treatment, right in

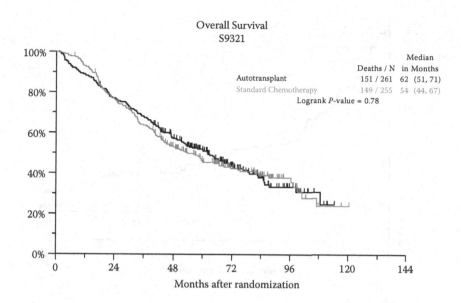

FIGURE 9.8
Survival distributions by randomized treatment arm for SWOG study S9321.

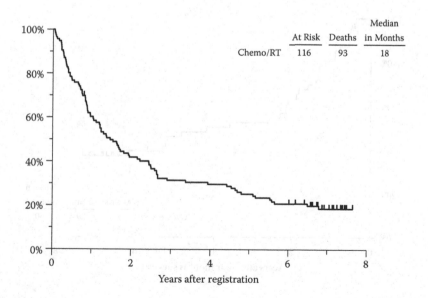

FIGURE 9.9
Survival distribution for all patients on SWOG lung cancer trial S8269.

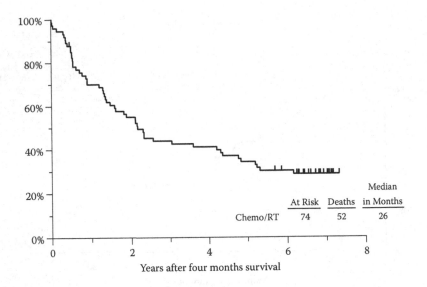

FIGURE 9.10
Survival distribution for patients on SWOG lung cancer trial S8269 with good performance status
and survival beyond 4 months.

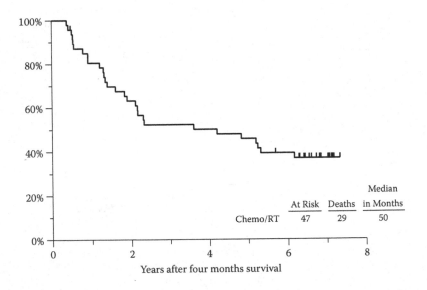

FIGURE 9.11
Survival distribution for patients on SWOG lung cancer trial S8269 with good performance status
and disease in complete response at 4 months.

the range of claimed benefit for high-dose therapy plus transplant. In this case further pilot studies were done which were not supportive of a randomized trial of high-dose therapy.

From these examples it should be clear that randomized trials to test new cancer treatments are indeed ethical. In fact, it might be unethical to claim superiority of such costly and toxic treatment as high-dose therapy and transplant without a randomized trial demonstrating efficacy.

9.3 Competing Risks

"Competing risks" refers to the problem of analyzing multiple possible failure types. For instance, patients being followed for relapse don't necessarily do so before they die, so relapse and death from other causes are the competing failure types for a disease-free survival endpoint. If particular sites of relapse are also of interest (e.g., local versus distant) then these are additional failure types. A common but misguided aim is to determine the effect of treatment on one endpoint (e.g., time to distant recurrence) after "eliminating" the risk of other endpoints (e.g., local recurrences and deaths due to other causes). Biology doesn't allow for elimination of outcomes without influence on other outcomes, and statistics can't either. A typical approach to estimating the distribution of time to a specific type of failure is to censor the observation at the time of any other type of failure if it occurs first, and calculate the Kaplan-Meier estimator from the resulting data. If outcomes were independent (meaning the probability of one outcome is the same regardless of the probability of other outcomes) there wouldn't be a major problem, but such independence is an unrealistic assumption. For instance, patients who have had a local relapse might then have a higher probability of distant relapse. Or, the same factors that result in a low probability of distant recurrence might influence the probability of death due to other causes as well. Sensitivity to chemotherapy might result in a higher probability of toxic death but a lower probability of distant recurrence. Alternatively, a poor immune system might result in a higher probability of both death and distant recurrence. Figure 7.1, which illustrates the potential bias when patients are lost to follow-up, applies here as well. Assume the loss to follow-up is due to the occurrence of a secondary endpoint. If patients who experience the secondary endpoint never experience the primary one, the top curve would apply. If patients who experience the secondary endpoint always experience the primary one immediately afterward, the bottom curve would apply. Censoring (middle curve) can result in bias in either direction. Endless combinations of relationships between endpoints can yield the same results. There is no way to tell which combination is correct without more complete information on all endpoints. There is no easy way to interpret such estimators.

Another approach sometimes taken is to follow patients for all types of endpoints until death or last known follow-up time. This approach is a slight improvement in that fewer endpoints have to be assumed independent. It does require that follow-up for all endpoints continues uniformly until death, which we find often not to be the case. Once a patient has metastatic disease, efforts to screen for—or at least to report—new local sites, new primaries, and other diseases are reduced.

The approach to estimation in the competing risks setting with perhaps the most support from statisticians is to decompose overall failure into cause-specific first failure components. In this approach no unrealistic assumptions are made in order to estimate a distribution in the absence of competing causes of failure. Instead, a sub-distribution function in the presence of all other failure types is estimated. This is also called (among other names) a *cumulative incidence* curve, although this term has also been used for other purposes. In this context, the cumulative incidence curve estimates at each time *t*, the probability of failing due to a specific cause by time *t* in the presence of competing failure types. Here's an example to illustrate. Suppose all 20 patients on a study of Treatment Q have failed at the following times for the following reasons.

Patient ID	Failure Time	Failure Type
1	1	death
2	11	death
3	2	distant
4	12	distant
5	3	death
6	13	local
7	4	local
8	14	death
9	5	distant
10	15	distant
11	6	distant
12	16	local
13	7	distant
14	17	death
15	8	distant
16	18	local
17	9	death
18	19	distant
19	10	distant
20	20	death

Figure 9.12 shows overall failure and cumulative incidences of the three failure types. For instance, the probability of failure at time 10 or before is estimated by the number of failures by time 10 over the total number on study, or 10/20. The probability of failure type "local" at time 10 or before is estimated as 1/20; the estimated probability of type "distant" is 6/20; the estimated probability of type "death" is 3/20. Since overall failure consists of the three types, the overall probability is the sum of the probabilities of the three types.

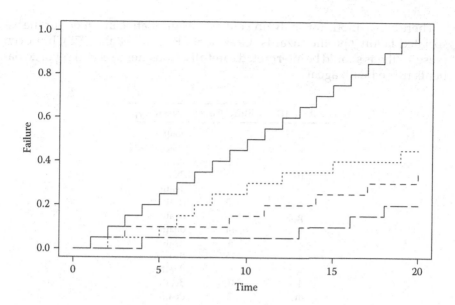

FIGURE 9.12
Overall failure (solid line) and cumulative incidences of three failure types: local recurrence (long-dashed line), distant recurrence (dotted line), deaths (short-dashed line).

With censored data the estimates are more complicated (Kalbfleisch and Prentice, 1980), but the idea of estimating the components of overall failure is the same. Gooley et al. (1999) have a nice description of the difference between the cumulative incidence and Kaplan-Meier (censored) approach. In Chapter 2 the Kaplan-Meier (K-M) estimator was described as a product

$$\left(\frac{n_1 - 1}{n_1}\right)\left(\frac{n_2 - 1}{n_2}\right)\ldots\left(\frac{n_i - 1}{n_i}\right),$$

where $n_1 \ldots n_i$ are the numbers of patients remaining at risk just before failure times $1 \ldots i$. Another way to describe the K-M estimator is to note that if there are N patients and no censoring, there is a drop of size $1/N$ at each time of failure. If there is censoring, then for the first patient censored, the assumption is made that failure for this patient should be just like failures for all other patients remaining alive at this time, so the K-M estimator divides up the $1/N$ drop for this patient among everyone left alive. For the next censored patient, $1/N$ plus whatever was allocated from the previous censored patient is divided up among everyone left alive at this time, and so on. For censorship due to the patient still being alive without failure, this is not unreasonable. With competing risks, however, the allocation generally doesn't make sense— death without relapse cannot be followed by a relapse. Rather than allocate the $1/N$ for a death without relapse to subsequent relapses (the K-M approach), the cumulative incidence approach recognizes that no relapse is possible and nothing is allocated.

There are methods for analyzing either the cumulative incidence or the associated failure-specific hazards (Gray, 1988; Prentice et al., 1978), but even these methods should be interpreted carefully. Consider a second set of 20 patients treated with agent X:

Patient ID	Failure Time	Failure Type
a	1	death
b	11	death
c	2	death
d	12	distant
e	3	death
f	13	death
g	4	death
h	14	death
i	5	death
j	15	distant
k	6	death
l	16	death
m	7	death
n	17	death
o	8	death
p	18	death
q	9	death
r	19	distant
s	10	distant
t	20	death

Figures 9.13–9.15 show the comparisons of cumulative incidence for local and distant recurrence and of death between the two data sets. Agent X appears to prevent local recurrence and to reduce distant recurrence. However, agent Q appears to prevent death. Is Q better? Or does Q cause recurrences so we don't see the deaths? The overall failure rate (time to local recurrence, distant recurrence, or death) is identical. A better endpoint for the choice of treatment would seem to be time to death (not recorded here for all patients).

Another approach to analysis (Prentice et al., 1978) is to compare cause-specific hazards (also called sub-hazards). A cause-specific hazard at time t is the rate of failure due to a specific cause given the patient is failure free at time t. The sum of all of the cause-specific hazards is the overall failure hazard (defined in Chapter 2). Just as for the overall hazard, differences in cause-specific hazards between two arms can be tested using a proportional hazards model (also defined in Chapter 2).

For this type of analysis, probabilities of cause-specific failure are not being compared, but rather the relative rate of failure. The two approaches are not equivalent. For instance, suppose the relapse hazard is the same on two arms, but the death hazard is higher on arm two. Comparing relapse probabilities will result in the conclusion that there are fewer relapses on arm two—since patients are dying faster on arm two, fewer are at risk for relapse so fewer relapses are seen. Comparing relapse hazards using a proportional hazards

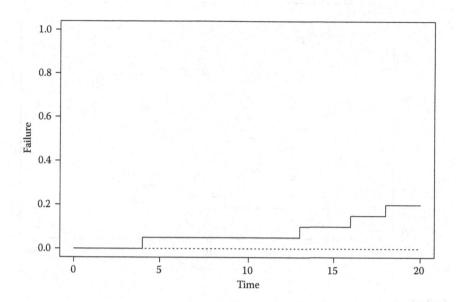

FIGURE 9.13
Cumulative incidence of local recurrence in two data sets, Q (solid line) and X (dotted line).

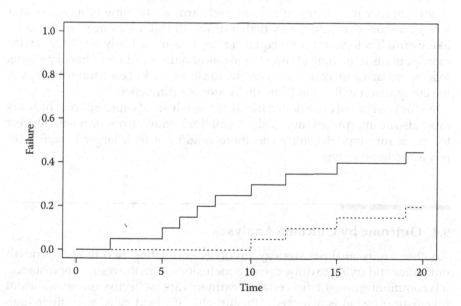

FIGURE 9.14
Cumulative incidence of distant recurrence in two data sets, Q (solid line) and X (dotted line).

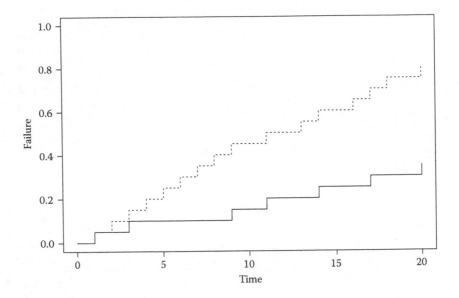

FIGURE 9.15
Cumulative incidence of death in two data sets, Q (solid line) and X (dotted line).

model, on the other hand, will result in a conclusion of no difference between the arms with respect to relapse. Roughly speaking, the computation looks at the number of patients at risk on each arm at the time of a failure and assigns a score depending on whether or not the failure came from the more likely arm. If relapse rates are equal, a relapse is more likely on the arm with more patients remaining at risk. As long as about the right number of patients relapse on each arm (conditional on the number at risk at each time of relapse), the comparison will not indicate that there is a difference.

As for analysis of cumulative incidence, analysis of cause-specific hazards must also be interpreted cautiously. A smaller hazard on one arm with respect to one failure type doesn't mean there might not be a larger hazard with respect to another type.

9.4 Outcome by Outcome Analyses

Another faulty analysis strategy involves correlating two time-dependent outcomes and trying to draw causal conclusions from the result. For instance, it is commonly thought that certain treatments are ineffective unless sufficient myelosuppression is achieved. (Presumably if blood cells, with their high turnover rate, are being killed, then so are cancer cells.) How would you prove this? A naive approach would be to look at minimum WBC achieved while on treatment versus survival time. Inevitably, low counts can be shown to be associated with longer survival. A little thought should reveal that the patients with the maximum number of shopping trips achieved in a week while on treatment live longer too, as do the ones who experience the most rainy days, the highest vitamin A levels, or the most mosquito bites in a month. Patients have to be alive for a measured variable to be observed; the longer a patient is alive the more often that variable is observed; the more often it's observed, the higher the maximum and the lower the minimum of the observations. Although reporting of this type of flawed analyses is less common than in the past, recent examples still occur, such as a report of association of rash with disease control in head and neck cancer patients treated with cetuximab (Vermorken et al., 2007).

9.4.1 Survival by Response Comparisons

Perhaps the longest standing misuse of statistics in oncology is the practice of comparing survival of responders to that of nonresponders. The belief appears to be that if responders live longer than nonresponders, then the treatment must be effective.

Of course, patients who respond live longer than ones who don't—patients have to live long enough to get a response, and those who die before evaluation of response are automatically classified as nonresponders. Suppose, for example, that everyone treated for six months gets a response at that time, and that response and survival are unrelated. In this case the responder versus nonresponder comparison is equivalent to comparing patients who are alive at 6 months versus ones who aren't. People alive at 6 months do indeed survive longer than ones who die before 6 months, but this observation has nothing to tell us about the effectiveness of treatment.

The comparison of responders to non-responders is completely analogous to the first published analysis of the potential benefit of heart transplantation (Clark et al., 1971), which compared the survival of those patients healthy enough to survive the waiting period for a donor heart, to that of patients who died before a new heart arrived. Most oncologists immediately recognize the latter as a fallacy, but the former persists. The fallacy has been given a mathematical formalization by Liu et al. (1993).

A better method of comparing responders with nonresponders is the "landmark" method (Anderson et al., 1983). In this approach response status is determined among living patients at a particular time (the landmark) after start of treatment. Then survival times subsequent to that time are compared. This eliminates the biases introduced by (1) defining early death as non-response and (2) by including the time before response as part of the survival time for responders (lead time bias). The cost of reducing the bias is loss of information from early deaths and classification of some late responders as nonresponders. Even though less biased than the simple comparison, the landmark method does not allow for a biologic interpretation of results. Responders might not live longer because they have achieved a response, but rather response might be a marker identifying patients who would have lived longer

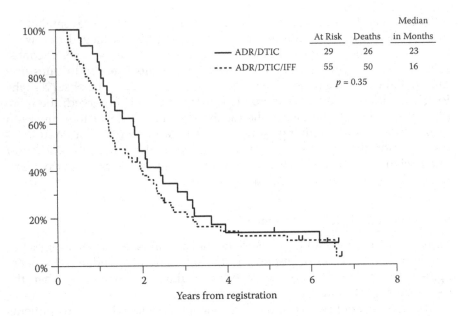

	At Risk	Deaths	Median in Months
—— ADR/DTIC	29	26	23
---- ADR/DTIC/IFF	55	50	16

$p = 0.35$

FIGURE 9.16
Survival distributions by treatment arm for responding patients on SWOG sarcoma trial S8616.

anyway—statistically there is no way to tell the difference. Still, it might be of clinical interest to know that among patients alive at 3 months, those who respond will generally live longer/the same/shorter than those who have not responded.

A related common, but misguided, analysis involves comparing treatments with respect to survival of responders or to duration of response. The reasoning behind such analyses seems to be that patients who do not respond to treatment receive minimal benefit from treatment, so responders are the primary group of interest. SWOG S8616 (Antman et al., 1993) provides a good example of the difficulties with this type of analysis. In this study, patients with advanced soft-tissue sarcoma were randomized to receive either Adriamycin plus DTIC (AD) or these same two agents plus Ifosfamide and Mesna (MAID). Response, time to failure, and survival were all endpoints of the study. In the next three paragraphs we demonstrate that AD is superior, that MAID is superior, and that AD and MAID are equivalent.

Figure 9.16 shows that survival of responders on AD is somewhat better than survival of responders on MAID. Under the assumption that patients who do not respond to treatment do not benefit from treatment, then the superior results of responders on AD suggests the superiority of AD.

Figure 9.17 shows that responders live longer than nonresponders on the study as a whole. The number of responders on MAID was 55/170 while the number on AD was 29/170. Clearly, since responders live longer and there were more responders on MAID, then MAID has been demonstrated to be superior.

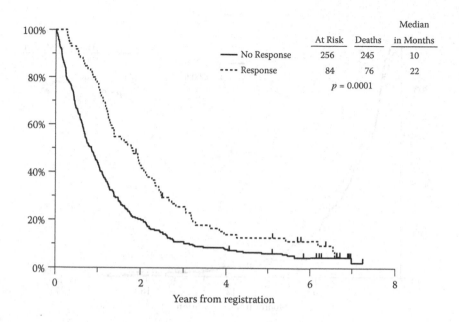

FIGURE 9.17
Survival distributions for responders versus nonresponders on SWOG sarcoma trial S8616.

Time to failure and survival curves for AD versus MAID are shown in Figures 9.18 and 9.19. The time to failure estimate is a little better on MAID, while survival is a little better on AD. Neither difference is significant. Neither regimen is shown to be preferable.

Which regimen should be recommended? MAID does result in more responses, although the ones gained over AD appear to be short (considering Figure 9.16). If the value of fleeting tumor shrinkage in the absence of survival benefit outweighs the substantial excess toxicity and cost due to Ifosfamide, then MAID should be recommended. If not, then AD would appear to be the better choice. Either way, it would have been a mistake to base a decision on Figure 9.16 or Figure 9.17—these confuse the interpretation of treatment differences more than they clarify.

9.4.2 "Dose Intensity" Analyses

Another variation on the theme of outcome by outcome analysis we have encountered is the analysis of survival according to planned or received total dose or dose intensity of treatment. These analyses usually are performed to show that more is better without the hassle of a clinical trial comparing doses. Famous examples are due to Hryniuk and Levine (1986), who observed a positive association of planned dose intensity with outcome in a collection of adjuvant studies in breast cancer, and Bonadonna and Valagussa (1981), who purport to demonstrate that high doses of received adjuvant chemotherapy are associated with improved survival, also in breast cancer.

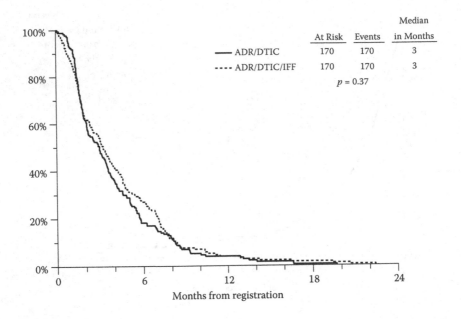

FIGURE 9.18
Time to treatment failure distributions by treatment arm for SWOG sarcoma trial S8616.

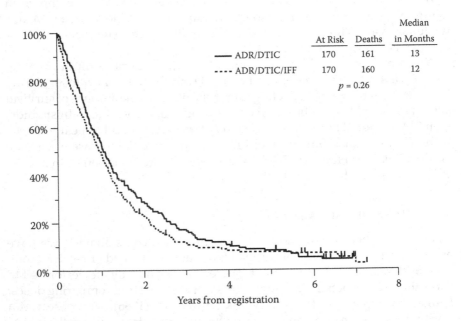

FIGURE 9.19
Survival distributions by treatment arm for SWOG sarcoma trial S8616.

Our own results with CMFVP noted above illustrate the difficulty in interpreting correlations of study outcomes with study characteristics such as planned dose intensity. Hryniuk and Levine hypothesized the importance of dose intensity based on (among other analyses) a plot of 3-year disease-free survival versus a weighted sum of the weekly doses of certain agents in the prescribed regimens of 27 arms from 17 adjuvant breast cancer studies. The apparent association was striking: disease-free survivals were 50%–57% for regimens of 0 intensity (no treatment); 53%–69% for intensities 0.1–0.5; 64%–86% for intensities 0.5–1. One of the problems with the analysis is that the studies compared may have differed with respect to factors not analyzed in the paper. As demonstrated by our series of CMFVP arms, factors other than dose may be having major influences on outcome. Despite a planned intensity of 1.0 for our CMFVP regimen, 3-year disease-free survivals on the five studies range from 58% to 73%, covering the middle 2/3 of survivals reported in the Hryniuk and Levine table. The arms in the table below 58% were all no treatment and single agent LPAM arms; the ones above 73% had planned intensities no greater than ours (lowest 0.71). It is not necessary to invoke intensity to explain the results of the table. A close look suggests an alternative explanation: no treatment or single agent LPAM are insufficient (50%–63%), and CMF-based regimens (64%–86%) are better than LF-based regimens (60%–69%). Henderson et al. (1988) discuss additional problems with the assumptions in the paper, such as the implied assumption that there were no time trends in breast cancer results (the more intense regimens were generally on studies conducted later in time).

Now consider the Bonadonna and Valagussa approach to showing high doses are beneficial, that of comparing patients who received higher doses on a trial with those who received lower doses. It should by now come as no surprise that analysis by dose received is as severely biased as the other outcome by outcome analyses described in this chapter. It can be conducted in ways that prove high doses, low doses, or intermediate doses are superior.

An example that illustrates the point clearly is taken from the cardiovascular literature (Coronary Drug Project Research Group, 1980). The Coronary Drug Project was a randomized double-blind, placebo controlled, five-arm trial of cholesterol-lowering agents. The 5-year mortality for 1103 men on one of the agents, clofibrate, was 20%, versus 21% in 2789 men on placebo, a disappointing result. A ray of hope might have been seen in the fact that clofibrate adherers had a substantially lower 5-year mortality than did poor adherers (15% for those who received $>= 80\%$ of protocol prescription versus 25% for those who received $< 80\%$). Perhaps at least the compliant patients benefitted from treatment. Alas, no. Compliance was even more strongly related to mortality in the placebo group: 15% mortality for $>= 80\%$ versus 28% for $< 80\%$. Evidently compliance functioned as a measure of good health.

Redmond et al. (1983) have an excellent cancer example. Doses received were collected for both arms of an adjuvant breast cancer trial of LPAM versus placebo. In the first comparison, the total received dose divided by the total planned dose was calculated for each patient and the following dose levels compared: level I $>=$ 85%, level II 65%–84%, level III $<$ 65%. Overall 5-year disease-free survival on the LPAM arm was 51%. The results for the three-dose levels were 69%, 67%, and 26% respectively, apparently a nice dose response. Disease-free survival in the placebo group was 46%, however. If we conclude that doses over 65% are beneficial, then must we also conclude that receiving $<$ 65% is harmful, since placebo was better than dose level III?

Most of the bias in this analysis comes from the fact that patients discontinued treatment if relapse occurred before the completion of the planned therapy, and therefore couldn't have had the highest doses. In effect, early failures were required to have low doses. This is seen clearly when the same analysis is done for placebo patients—an even better dose response is observed! Five-year disease-free survivals for patients who took $>=$ 85%, 65%–84%, and $<$65% of placebo were 69%, 43%, 12%. Patients did not fail because their received dose was low, but received a low dose because they failed.

No method eliminates all the biases. The next comparison in the Redmond paper shows how another approach fails. To reduce the bias in the first method, it might seem logical to calculate instead the total dose received divided by the dose planned prior to the time of failure. Unfortunately, this isn't much better—the bias switches the other way. Patients who fail late are more likely to have received low protocol doses, since they have had more time to experience toxicity requiring dose reductions, or to become noncompliant. For LPAM, 5-year disease-free survivals by dose levels I, II, and III defined this way are 47%, 59%, 55%; for placebo they are 47%, 43%, and 60%.

The third method discussed is a landmark method, similar to that described for response. The landmark chosen was 2 years (the length of prescribed treatment) and survival after 2 years among those who had not yet failed was compared as a function of dose received. Although the differences were not significant, middle doses were the winners for this analysis. The first 2 years of information is a lot to ignore, however, so one final method was used, a time-dependent Cox model (Cox, 1972). This can be thought of as a way to switch to a new landmark at each failure time. While quite sophisticated statistically, this final method still has problems: the placebo dose was again significantly associated with survival.

Dose analysis problems start the instant one tries to define received dose intensity. "The amount of drug administered per unit time" is a common definition of intensity, but it is not complete unless a single agent is administered at the same dose at the same unit interval for the same number of intervals in every patient. If there are multiple agents, a method must be devised for combining agents into a single intensity measure; the possibilities for weighting schemes are infinite. If doses are modified over time, then there is no single amount per unit time; some sort of average must be devised. If treatment is given according to an interval other than the unit interval, then again there is no single amount per unit time. If treatment duration is variable, then "amount per unit time" is a function not only of unit doses, but also of how many units. Should "per unit time" be calculated during the time the patient received treatment, during the time the patient was supposed to receive treatment, or during some fixed interval?

SWOG study S7827 again provides an example. As noted in Chapter 6, this trial compared 1 year versus 2 years of SWOG standard CMFVP in node-positive receptor-negative breast cancer patients. The regimen consisted of daily administration of cyclophosphamide (ctx), weekly administration of methotrexate (mtx) and 5-fluorouracil (5-FU), plus short-term vincristine (vcr) and prednisone. How should intensity be summarized?

First consider how to define interval intensity. Summaries per week are more common than per day, but note that in choosing a weekly interval the assumption is being made that daily doses of cyclophosphamide are equivalent to the same total dose given weekly. Then consider how to combine weekly doses into a single measure. Weighting according to the content of the Cooper et al. (1979) CMF regimen is typical, i.e., ctx/560+ mtx/17+5FU/294. Note this weighting makes the assumption that 1 mg/m^2 of single agent mtx, 33 of ctx, and 17 of 5FU are all interchangeable, and that vcr and prednisone contribute nothing to intensity. If we want to add contributions for vcr and prednisone, how to do so is problematic since these agents aren't given as long as the others. Should the 10 weeks of vcr be averaged over the year treatment is given? Should the intensity measure be changed after 10 weeks?

A large number of fairly arbitrary assumptions and decisions have to be made to define interval intensity. Another set of assumptions and decisions have to be made in order to combine all the intervals for a patient into a single measure. Is a simple average of unit intensities over the course of treatment a sufficient summary? If so, then the assumption is being made that 6 months of 95% doses followed by 6 months of 5% is equivalent to the reverse. If a patient on the 1-year arm and the 2-year arm has identical doses for the first year, should the intensity summary be the same? If yes, then the assumption has to be made that doses in the 2-year contribute nothing to intensity. If no, and weekly intensities are averaged over the planned course of treatment, then if the patient on the 2-year arm quits after 1 year (recall from Chapter 6 that compliance with 2 years was poor) intensity will be one-half the intensity of the 1-year patient despite identical treatment.

Better statistical methods will never yield results that answer the question of whether more myelosuppressive, more responsive or more intense regimens are more effective. Many factors associated with survival are also associated with other outcomes. For instance, in the SWOG study just discussed, we found menopausal status and age to be associated with dose. (Premenopausal patients received the highest doses, post 60 and older the lowest, and post less than 60 middle range doses.) It might be possible to adjust for the few factors we know about, but most factors are unmeasured or unknown or both. Part or all of any association (or lack of association) of survival with attained dose or any other outcome may well be explained by these other factors.

Considering all the biases in analyzing survival by dose, and the fact that "intensity" can't even be defined sensibly, we hope you are persuaded that dose intensity analyses have no useful scientific interpretation. The way to answer questions about dose intensity is through randomized trials!

9.5 Subset Analyses

The temptation to go beyond a simple treatment comparison of the primary endpoint is almost irresistible. If the study is negative overall, it would be nice if there were some subset of patients (women, good performance status, young, etc.) for which a benefit associated with the new treatment could be shown. Similarly, if in the overall comparison there is an advantage for the new treatment over the standard, it is of interest to find subsets for which the advantage is greater, and some for which it is not beneficial at all. The problem with such good intentions is that most such subset analyses arrive at incorrect conclusions. See, for example, Rothwell (2005) for a good discussion of subset analysis issues, recommendations, and examples—including the classic astrologic sign example from the 17,187 patient ISIS-2 trial (ISIS-2 Collaborative Group, 1988; Collins and MacMahon, 2001) in which subset analyses showed that Libra and Gemini patients did not benefit from aspirin treatment while all others did.

When subset analyses are done, a common practice is to report only those results that yielded a positive result, giving the reader no idea of how many subsets were investigated. This poor reporting of subset results was studied by Wang et al. (2007). Of 97 randomized trials published in the *New England Journal of Medicine* from July 2005 to June 2006 only 25 had consistent reporting of all subsets tested and only 2 of the 15 reporting dissimilar subset results had cautions about interpretation. In 1989 the Mayo Clinic published a study that demonstrated a survival advantage for the combination of 5-FU and levamisole over observation after surgery for patients with Dukes' C colon cancer (Laurie et al., 1989). The authors then looked at subsets of patients to see whether some groups benefitted from therapy more than others. They found that adjuvant therapy was most effective for males, and for older patients. A large confirmatory trial was undertaken, involving several groups, with the Southwest Oncology Group as the statistical center. The overall result was consistent with the earlier trial: patients with Dukes' C colon cancer treated with 5-FU plus levamisole after surgery had a better survival outcome than did patients on observation (Moertel et al., 1990). However, when we looked at the same subsets as in the Mayo study, we found that adjuvant therapy was most effective for females, and for younger patients: the exact opposite! Figure 9.20 illustrates the results for males.

We previously reviewed eight trials testing the efficacy of infusion of 5-FU into the portal vein following surgery for colorectal cancer (Crowley, 1994). Three trials were reported as positive for portal vein infusion therapy, 5 as negative. Among the positive trials, therapy was found to be more effective in Dukes' C patients in one trial and in Dukes, B in another; a formal statistical

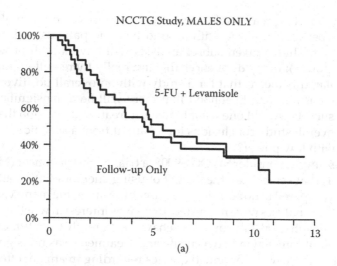

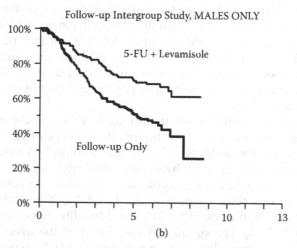

FIGURE 9.20
Subset analysis of males from: (a) original study; and (b) confirmatory study.

test of whether treatment results varied by subset was negative in the third trial. Among the negative trials, positive subsets were found for Dukes' C patients in one, for all those surviving 6 months in another, and for Dukes' C patients surviving 3 years in a third. No subset differences were found in the other two trials. The overall benefit of portal vein infusion is in doubt (and is the subject of a published meta-analysis—see Chapter 10); the subset analyses are clearly noise.

Why do such subset analyses so often go wrong? The reasons are simple. Most cancer clinical trials do not have adequate sample size to have a good chance of detecting reasonable treatment differences in the overall comparison, so a particular subset, with around half the patients, will have even lower power. Thus a given subset analysis will have a high false-negative rate (low power); many differences that are really there will go undetected. In particular, this means that for a study with an overall positive treatment result, there is a strong likelihood that there will be a nonsignificant result for some subsets. Would one want to make a treatment decision that differed from the overall study conclusions for a patient from a specific subset, based on a test with low power?

As an example, consider SWOG S9008, a trial in gastric cancer (Macdonald et al., 2001) that established the benefit of using chemoradiation after gastric resection compared to no additional treatment. Among the many variables for which subset analyses were requested, there was interest in whether tumors of the gastro-esophageal (GE) junction behaved differently from tumors of other sites. A test of interaction between site and treatment was not significant. In spite of this, there were continued queries regarding treatment effects within the subset of patients with GE junction tumors. However, of the 553 eligible patients on this trial, only 20% had tumors of the GE junction. We determined that based on these numbers, the power to detect the study-specific hazard ratio in this subset was approximately 40%. Would we want to publish a result that had such a poor chance of demonstrating the clinical result? Based on the nonsignificant interaction, and such low power, we did not pursue further exploration in this subset.

Fleming (1995) performed a simulation study to assess the reliability of subset analyses when the overall treatment effect was positive. This simulation, based on data from a double-blind, placebo controlled trial of dornase alfa in 968 patients with cystic fibrosis, estimated false-negative rates when only three covariates were the subject of subset analyses. The covariates were age (categorized into three levels, representing 50%, 20%, and 30% of the population, respectively); sex (50%, 50%), and baseline forced vital capacity (FVC- 40%, 30%, 30%). The simulation assumed that the overall treatment effect was constant across all subsets of patients, and 1000 trials were generated, randomly assigning patients to different covariate levels for each trial. In 67% of the trials, the treatment was estimated to be of no benefit, or even harmful in at least one level of one of the three covariates. This false-negative rate would have been even higher if the number of subsets tested had been increased.

Subset analyses suffer from more than low power. When the overall test of treatment does not conclude a benefit of one treatment over the other, subset analyses are viewed as a way to save something from the trial, or at the very least, make the manuscript more interesting. Once one starts down the road of doing subset analyses, it is very difficult to stop. After looking within races, sexes, stages, performance status categories, histologies, tumor grades, *ad infinitum*, something is bound to show up as being statistically significant just by chance (this is the multiple comparison problem considered in the context of multi-arm trials in Chapter 6, interim analyses in Chapter 6, and exploratory analyses in Chapter 10). Multiple subset analyses are subject to a high false-positive rate; many of the differences detected are not really there.

The combined problems of poor power for real differences, and high false-positive rates means that almost all subset analyses are wrong. Thus, all subset analyses must be confirmed in subsequent trials before they can be believed.

What can be done to minimize these difficulties, given the imperative to explore data for clues? First, understand that if results in a given subset are important and likely to be different, separate trials should be designed, or a given trial should be designed with adequate power for that subset analysis, including proper attention to the multiple comparison problem. Second, understand that stratification for the purpose of balance at randomization does not justify subset analyses by stratification factors. Such analyses are still subject to a high false-negative rate due to inadequate sample size, and a high false-positive rate unless each comparison is done at a very low significance level or using a model that allows first for a formal statistical test of whether treatment differences vary by subset. Third, be aware that subset analyses are exploratory and hypothesis generating, and thus not to be given nearly the same credibility as the overall treatment comparison. Any presentation or publication of results should make clear which results can be taken as definitive and which as exploratory; as a rule, the overall treatment comparison of the primary endpoint is definitive (in a well designed trial); the rest is speculative.

9.6 Surrogate Endpoints

Survival is the preferred primary endpoint in cancer clinical trials, being both objective and of obvious validity. In certain adjuvant trials (in breast cancer, for example) it is not practical to insist on survival as the primary endpoint, because not enough events will be observed in a realistic time frame; thus disease-free survival is used instead. It could be said in such cases that disease-free survival, which is known sooner but is somewhat subjective and does not perfectly reflect long-term outcome, is used as a replacement or surrogate for survival (which is usually an important secondary endpoint). A more common use of the term surrogate endpoint is for very short-term outcomes such as tumor response, tumor markers in cancer prevention trials, and CD4 count in AIDS trials. The motivation for the use of such surrogate endpoints is obvious: we'd like to be able to make decisions about treatment efficacy with smaller sample sizes and without having to wait for the real endpoint to occur.

A few examples should suffice to give pause about the use of surrogate endpoints. We have already seen in the sarcoma trial of AD versus MAID that a higher tumor response rate does not necessarily translate into better survival. The same phenomenon occurred with 5-FU and leucovorin in advanced colon cancer. A review of several trials (Advanced Colorectal Meta-Analysis Project, 1992) indicated that response was strikingly improved with the combination ($p < 0.0001$) but that there was no effect on survival ($p = 0.57$). The opposite can also happen: Gil Deza et al. (1996) reported a survival advantage for vinorelbine and cisplatin over vinorelbine alone in patients with advanced non-small cell lung cancer ($p = 0.02$) but no response advantage ($p = 0.97$).

In the Cardiac Arrythmia Suppression Trial (Echt et al., 1991) in patients having a recent myocardial infarction, ecainide, and flecainide were compared to placebo for survival post MI. These agents reduce ventricular arrhythmias, which are a risk factor for subsequent sudden death. Many argued that a placebo-controlled trial was not only unnecessary but unethical, since an effect on the surrogate endpoint of ventricular arrhythmias had already been established. The trial was done anyway, and with over 1500 randomized patients the startling result was that the drugs more than doubled the death rate relative to placebo (the rate was more than tripled for causes due to arrhythmias).

From the field of AIDS research, a trial conducted in the United States by the Aids Clinical Trials Group (Volberding et al., 1990) testing the effect of zidovudine for slowing disease progression in asymptomatic HIV-infected people was stopped early for positive results based on interim analysis of this surrogate endpoint (progression). A later trial done in Europe (Concorde Coordinating Committee, 1994) found that with longer follow-up the effect on the surrogate was lost, and no effect on survival was found. (See DeMets et al., 1995, for a discussion of the first trial from the point of view of the data monitoring committee.)

Prentice (1989) has given mathematical conditions that would permit the use of surrogate endpoints. In order to guarantee that the inference from the surrogate is the same as would be obtained from the primary endpoint, it is necessary to assume that all the information on treatment differences is contained in the surrogate, clearly an impossible case. Buyse and Molenberghs (1998) suggest a more practical perspective, defining individual surrogacy to mean there is a strong association between the true endpoint and the surrogate after adjustment for treatment, and population surrogacy to mean the effect of treatment on the surrogate predicts the effect of treatment on the true endpoint. With a sufficient number of patients, individual surrogacy is relatively easy to demonstrate or disprove, but unfortunately this does not allow conclusions about population surrogacy. For this, a sufficient number of randomized studies is required to demonstrate a high correlation between the difference in the surrogate by treatment arm and the difference in the true endpoint by treatment arm. For example, Sargent et al. (2005), analyzed 18 randomized adjuvant studies with 43 treatment arms and 20,898 patients in order to demonstrate that disease-free survival (DFS) is a suitable endpoint for assessing treatment effect in colon cancer patients in place of survival. They examined individual level, arm level and study level associations of DFS and survival, noting high correlations for each. Most importantly, the correlation between DFS and survival hazard ratios was 0.92, and for 23 of

25 comparisons, the logrank tests of DFS and of survival provided the same conclusion. The analysis was persuasive, but not ideal in that DFS is still a long-term endpoint. Of course in most settings such extensive information is not available and surrogacy cannot be verified.

Another possible approach to the problem is to model the association of the surrogate with the primary endpoint as you go along and to use the information gained to strengthen inferences on the primary endpoint. It turns out that the information gained is highly dependent on being able to model the relationships correctly. Even the enthusiasts of this approach agree that it doesn't help unless there is a very high correlation between the primary and surrogate endpoint. Hsieh et al. (1983) investigate various realistic models of the relationship between disease progression and death, and find that incorporating progression into the analysis of survival adds little strength to the inference, even when the correct model is assumed.

The inescapable conclusion is that trials must be designed to detect differences in real clinical endpoints of interest. Surrogates are most useful in the context of Phase II trials, to screen agents for further randomized testing of effects on primary endpoints.

10

Exploratory Analyses

In real life research is dependent on the human capacity for making predictions
that are wrong and on the even more human gift for bouncing back to try again.

—Lewis Thomas (1983)

10.1 Introduction

Cancer clinical trials should be designed primarily to get precise answers
to important questions about the efficacy of treatment. However, there is
considerable interest in also trying to learn something about the underlying
biology of the disease during the course of a trial or a series of trials. Data
are collected on patient demographics, tumor characteristics, and various
other host factors in an attempt to understand which variables are useful in
predicting patient outcome, both for use in subsequent trials and in explaining
the results of a given trial. As opposed to the definitive treatment comparison,
these statistical analyses are exploratory, serving to generate and not prove
hypotheses. The general kinds of questions addressed include the following:
What are the important prognostic factors? How can they be used to in the
design of future trials? Are there identifiable subsets of patients that do so
well that there is little room for improvements in treatment? Are there subsets
that do so poorly that much more aggressive strategies should be devised?

We illustrate some aspects of these exploratory analyses using data from
a SWOG trial of multiple myeloma (SWOG S8229, Salmon et al., 1990) with
survival as the outcome of interest, but the issues are of course more general.
More detailed analyses of these data are given in Crowley et al. (1995), and
Crowley et al. (1997).

10.2 Some Background and Notation

Patients with multiple myeloma have a predominant clone of affected plasma
cells and thus a compromised immune system. They are thus subject to various infections, and also often have kidney trouble and bone lesions and

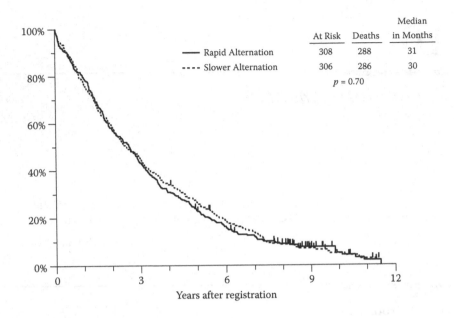

	At Risk	Deaths	Median in Months
—— Rapid Alternation	308	288	31
- - - Slower Alternation	306	286	30

$p = 0.70$

FIGURE 10.1
Survival distributions by treatment in SWOG myeloma trial S8229.

fractures. The introduction of therapy with melphalan and prednisone in the 1950s increased the median survival for patients with this disease from less than 1 year to 30–36 months. The course of the disease is extremely variable but most patients eventually die of myeloma or its complications. Consequently, there is an interest in understanding which factors at diagnosis predict survival, and in developing staging systems that could be used in stratification or in defining subsets for differing therapeutic interventions.

SWOG S8229 was designed to test whether two four-drug combinations (vincristine, melphalan, cyclophosphamide, prednisone; vincristine, BCNU, Adriamycin, prednisone) should be given in rapid succession or in a more slowly alternating fashion. There was evidence that cancer cells resistant to one combination would be susceptible to treatment with the other, and some theory (the Goldie-Coldman hypothesis, Goldie et al., 1982) that such non-cross-resistant regimens should be given as close in time as possible for maximum effect. We randomized 614 patients to the two regimens and found virtually no difference in survival (Figure 10.1). SWOG S8624 compared one of the arms from SWOG S8229 with two other regimens containing more steroids, with modest differences in favor of the latter two arms.

A staging system previously in common use was due to Durie and Salmon (1975), and is based on a quantification of the number of tumor cells (stages I–III) and a classification of kidney function (A, B). This system was used to stratify the patients in SWOG S8229 (I-II versus IIIA versus IIIB, Figure 10.2).

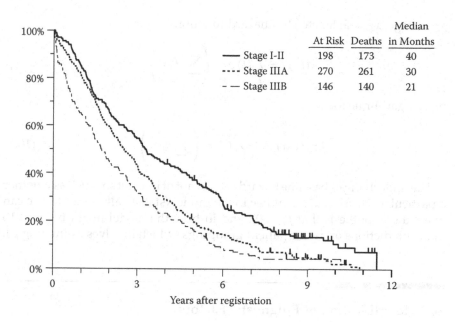

FIGURE 10.2
Survival distributions by Durie-Salmon stage in SWOG myeloma trial S8229.

Besides Durie-Salmon stage, information routinely collected on the myeloma prestudy includes albumin, creatinine, age, race, myeloma subtype (light and heavy chain proteins involved), and serum β_2 microglobulin (sb2m), a prognostic factor first identified in the 1980s (Norfolk et al., 1980; Battaille et al., 1983) which rises with either increasing tumor burden or decreased kidney function. We wanted to know if these variables predicted survival, and if we could derive a more predictive and reproducible staging system than the Durie-Salmon system.

Statistically, these questions can be addressed within the framework of Cox, or proportional hazards, regression, introduced in Chapter 2. (Analogously, other measured variables not subject to censoring can be explored using ordinary multiple linear regression or any of its generalizations, and dichotomized categorical variables can be explored using a model relating probabilities to covariates, such as logistic regression.) Since the methods are exploratory, there is more of an emphasis on looking at data graphically to find relationships, but some aspects of formal hypothesis testing and estimation are usually employed (subject to caveats regarding multiple comparisons and post-hoc fallacies). With survival analysis the fact that some survival times may be censored makes the graphical aspects all the more challenging.

Recall from Chapter 2 that the proportional hazards model characterizes a patient's hazard or risk of dying as a function of time and measured variables of interest. Thus the model states that a patient with covariates x ($x_1 = $ age,

$x_2 = $ stage, $x_3 = $ sb2m etc.) has hazard function

$$\lambda(t, x) = \lambda_0(t) \exp \left(\sum_i \beta_i x_i \right),$$

or in logarithmic form

$$\ln \lambda(t, x) = \ln \lambda_0(t) + \left(\sum_i \beta_i x_i \right). \tag{10.1}$$

The underlying or baseline hazard $\lambda_0(t)$ is not of interest so much as whether a particular covariate x_i should be in the model (statistically, whether we can reject the hypothesis that β_i is 0); and in how the model might be used to make predictions or derive patient groupings (which involves estimating β).

10.3 Identification of Prognostic Factors

In principle the answer to the question of whether, say, sb2m is an important prognostic factor can be answered very simply by the statistician: fit a Cox model and test whether the coefficient associated with sb2m is 0 or not (the test statistic is a generalization of the logrank test). In practice, there are a host of difficulties and complications that the user of such models needs to appreciate. First, there is the issue of the scale of measurement. A covariate like sb2m is continuous: should it be used as a continuous variable in the regression modelling, or dichotomized or otherwise turned into a categorical variable? If continuous, should it be in the original scale or some other scale (e.g., logarithmic)? If categorical, how are the cutpoints of the categories to be chosen? Second, is it of primary interest to see if sb2m is prognostic at all (in a univariate model, with no other variables present), or prognostic even in the presence of other variables (in a model with multiple other variables, i.e., a multivariate model). If the latter, how is this multivariate model developed, from the literature or the data at hand? If from the data, there is the question of the scale of measurement for each of the other variables, the question of whether derived variables are considered (e.g., products of two variables), and the question of how a final model is chosen from among countless possibilities even given answers to the other questions (step-down, step-up, stepwise, all subset selection, etc.—see Draper and Smith, 1968 for a general discussion of these methods). We address each of these areas in turn.

10.3.1 Scale of Measurement

As usual, there are trade-offs regarding the choice of a scale of measurement for a putative prognostic factor. The simplest choice for a continuous covariate is to use the measurements as recorded and ask whether the coefficient is significant in a Cox regression model. This is also the most powerful, in the sense of detecting an effect if there really is one, provided the assumed model is correct. However, there is little likelihood that any regression model is exactly correct, and it is well known that a few extreme values of the covariate can greatly affect the results of a regression analysis. Transformations of the covariate (e.g., by taking logs) can reduce the dependence on extreme values, but the choice of a particular transformation can be problematic. Covariates can be categorized to create two or more groups, but the choice of boundaries for the groupings can be difficult (possibilities include using previously published values, using the median or other percentiles of the observed covariate distribution, or using data-driven cutpoints). We illustrate these choices using sb2m as a potential predictor of survival in our sample of myeloma patients treated on SWOG S8229.

The covariate sb2m was recorded for 548 of the 614 eligible patients on study. It is typical to have some missing values of a covariate, for various reasons. Such missing data can jeopardize an analysis of prognostic factors, especially if the reasons for missing data are related to the variables under study. The best approach is to minimize such missingness through protocol requirements (sb2m was not an eligibility criterion for S8229); a distant second best is to investigate whether the other covariates and the outcome of interest vary depending on whether data are missing on a particular covariate. Figure 10.3 shows that the patients with and without available sb2m measurements have roughly comparable survival, a reassuring but not conclusive observation.

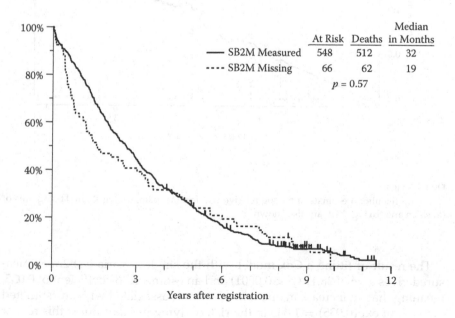

FIGURE 10.3
Survival distributions by presence of sb2m in SWOG myeloma trial S8229.

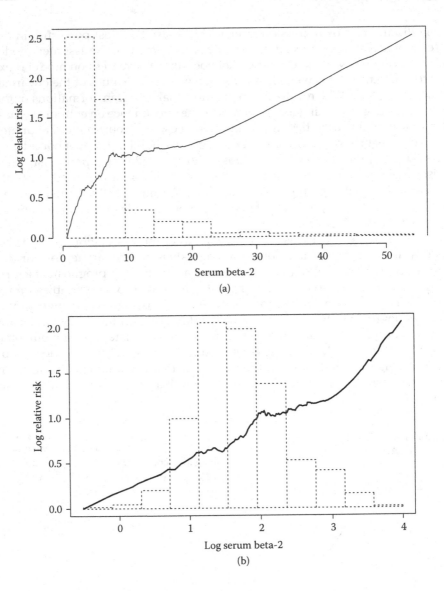

FIGURE 10.4
Local full likelihood estimate of the log relative risk for: (a) sb2m; (b) log sb2m. Histograms of
(a) sb2m and (b) log sb2m are also shown.

The result of fitting a Cox model with the single covariate sb2m as measured gives a χ^2 of 38.11 ($p < 0.0001$) and an estimated β coefficient of 0.035,
meaning that an increase in one unit of sb2m is associated with an estimated
increase of $\exp(0.035) = 1.035$ in the risk of dying per day. But is this real or
artifactual? Figure 10.4a shows the distribution of sb2m values, which as is
typical for laboratory measurements is highly skewed, with a few large values

that have a great deal of influence on the fit of the Cox regression model. Figure 10.4b shows that the distribution of the log of sb2m has fewer extreme values. Fitting log sb2m in a Cox model gives a χ^2 of 36.45 ($p < 0.0001$) and an estimated coefficient of 0.360, which means an estimated increase in risk of dying of $\exp(0.360) = 1.434$ for a unit increase in log sb2m. But which model is better? Statistical techniques now exist for estimating the regression relationship (the summation in equation 10.1) without assuming it has the linear form $\sum \beta_i x_i$ (Tibshirani and Hastie, 1987; Gentleman and Crowley 1991a). One such fit is shown in 10.4a for sb2m, suggesting a highly nonlinear relationship. A similar fit for log sb2m is given in 10.4b; the latter relationship is more nearly linear, indicating that using $x = \log$ sb2m in the Cox model with the linear form $\sum \beta_i x_i$ is more appropriate than using $x =$ sb2m without such a transformation.

It would seem wise in any case to step back from fitting a regression model and take a look at the data. When plotting survival data, however, the censored data points can distort the message that complete data would provide. Figure 10.5 is a scatterplot of survival and log sb2m, with censored observations plotted with open circles, uncensored ones with closed circles. It is difficult to discern trends in the scatterplot by itself, both because of the censoring and because of the inherent variability of the data. Merely superimposing a straight line fit would not be appropriate, because some of the data are censored. However, one can use techniques to fit a curve through the "center" of the data, where for a given value of log sb2m those patients with nearby covariate values are grouped and the median survival or other percentiles of the distribution are calculated (Gentleman and Crowley, 1991b).

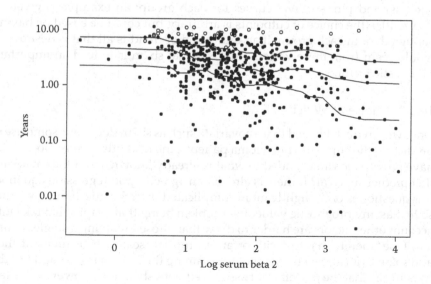

FIGURE 10.5
Scatterplot of survival versus log sb2m with smoothed quartile estimators.

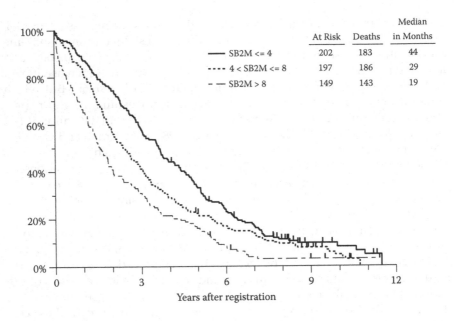

	At Risk	Deaths	Median in Months
—— SB2M <= 4	202	183	44
···· 4 < SB2M <= 8	197	186	29
– – SB2M > 8	149	143	19

FIGURE 10.6
Survival distributions by values of sb2m in SWOG myeloma trial S8229.

Figure 10.5 shows these "running quantile" plots for the median and the 75th and 25th percentiles, indicating a decrease in survival with increasing values of log sb2m. An even simpler approach would be to categorize sb2m into a few groups (three or more is recommended, depending on how much data one has) and plot survival curves for each group; an example is given in Figure 10.6 (the choice of cutpoints is arbitrary, but could be based on having enough data in each group, if an indication of trend is all that is desired). It would seem from these various analyses that sb2m is indeed an important prognostic factor.

10.3.2 Choice of Model

Once we have established that a covariate such as sb2m does have some use in predicting the survival of myeloma patients, the next question is: Does sb2m have prognostic value, added to what is already known about the covariates that predict survival? If there is already an agreed upon regression equation, this question is only slightly more complicated than the question of whether sb2m has any prognostic value (the problem being that graphs that take into account other factors are harder to draw than those involving a single covariate). One "merely" has to decide on an appropriate scale of measurement, then add sb2m to an agreed upon model containing the known factors and test the hypothesis that the β coefficient associated with sb2m is 0. However, it is fair to say that there is no situation in cancer research where there is complete agreement on which prognostic factors are important, much less on the form of the model containing those factors. One is thus left with having to decide on the scale of measurement for each known factor and on whether derived variables such as products are to be included in a model before even addressing the question of the added value of sb2m. Often the situation is even more complicated than that, the question being not does this covariate add information but rather, which of dozens of candidate variables are "the" important prognostic factors (and which is the most important, which is next, etc.).

There is an extensive statistical literature on fitting such regression models, especially but not exclusively in the context of uncensored data. Excellent recent reviews of regression methods with censored data are given in Schumacher et al. (2006), Ulm et al. (2006), Thall and Estey (2001), and Sasieni and Winnett (2001). There are at least as many strategies as there are statisticians. One can step up, in the sense that "all" variables (and derived variables such as products? products of three or more variables? different scales for each variable?) are considered by themselves one by one, in univariate models, and the most statistically significant is chosen in the first step. The remaining variables are then considered as to whether they add to the first, etc. Or, one can step down, first fitting a model with all possible variables and then seeing which can be eliminated as least significant. (This approach is rarely possible due to the large number of candidate variables and the fact that few patients will have complete data on all of them). Or, one can adopt a stepwise strategy, stepping up but seeing at each step if any previously included variable can now be excluded. Yet another approach is to select the "best" from all possible models, something conceivable only in statistical textbooks.

A related technique to Cox regression modelling is the use of neural networks (or neural nets), which are really no more than complicated regression models hidden behind the language of artificial intelligence. An example using the data from SWOG myeloma study S8229 is given by Faraggi, LeBlanc, and Crowley (2001). The results are not much different from the use of Cox regression, provided one keeps the neural net to a manageable number of parameters, and includes product terms (also called interactions) in the Cox model. The disadvantage of neural nets is that the results are difficult to interpret in terms of the effects of the original variables.

Apart from all the more subjective modelling decisions, there is the fact that a multitude of formal statistical tests are being done. This multiple comparison issue was also raised in Chapters 3 and 6, but it is an even more severe problem in the present context. (Should each test be done at the 5% level? The 0.5% level? Is there a level for each test that is small enough to protect against making false positive statements?) This is not science, and perhaps not art. Many of us have heard confident proclamations that such and so variable is important in multivariate analysis; perhaps now you have an appreciation of the fact that this translates to "my statistician and I think we have something here." In the case of sb2m, we think we have something. It has been found to be important by others. It is important in our data in univariate analyses, using various scales of measurement. It is the first variable entered in the step-wise modelling we have done. And, "it is statistically significant in a multivariate analysis, after adjusting for other known prognostic factors ($p <$ 0.001)."

10.4 Forming Prognostic Groups

Given an agreed upon Cox regression model (!) one can make predictions about the survival of patients with given prognostic factors. While it should be clear that this cannot be done with any precision, one might use a Cox regression model to group patients into broad prognostic categories or stages (based on deciles, quartiles etc. of patient values of the regression function βx, or by assigning patients into categories based on how many of the good or bad values of prognostic variables they had). While such staging schemes have proven useful, they are difficult to interpret. A more direct technique called recursive partitioning may have some advantages in this regard.

Recursive partitioning can be described as follows. Each candidate prognostic variable is used to divide the patients into two groups, based on all possible cutpoints for that variable. The best (over all variables and all cutpoints) such split is found, where "best" might be defined as maximizing the logrank statistic between the two groups (Ciampi et al., 1986; Segal, 1988). This rule is then applied to each of the resulting two groups, and then recursively to the data until there are a large number of groups, each containing only a small number of patients. Next, there are rules that allow one to combine groups and choose the best staging system. There are several potential advantages to this approach to forming prognostic groups. One is that the scale of measurement is not an issue, except that a monotonic relationship must be assumed between covariates and survival (e.g., survival tends to go down as sb2m goes up). Another is that the resulting groups are easily described (a good prognosis group being those with low sb2m and high albumin, for example). In addition, there are built-in mechanisms (sample re-use, such as cross-validation, Breiman et al., 1984) that try to minimize the extent to which one is fooled by making multiple comparisons. However, there are still difficulties, among them the fact that use of another statistic besides the logrank test results in different groupings, and that the precise split points for a given set of data are unlikely to be duplicated in the next.

Figure 10.7 is a plot of the value of the logrank statistic as a function of the value of the covariate, for several covariates in the SWOG S8229 data set. The best split into two groups based on the logrank statistic is for the covariate sb2m, at a value of 5.4 nanograms per milliliter; the Chi-squared statistic for this split is 38 ($p < 0.0001$) but this needs to be adjusted for the fact that it is the maximum logrank statistic over all possible cutpoints. The p-value adjusted for multiple comparisons is still highly significant (see LeBlanc and Crowley, 1993, for a discussion of the details of the adjustment procedure).

A regression tree based on our recursive partitioning algorithm (LeBlanc and Crowley, 1992) using all candidate variables is given in Figure 10.8. The

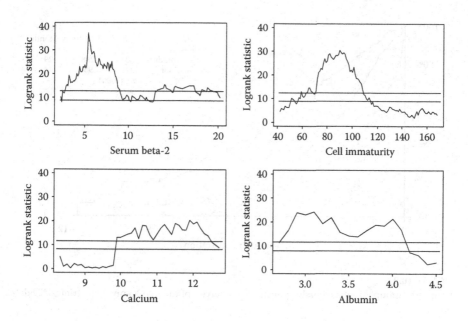

FIGURE 10.7

The logrank statistic as a function of several covariates in the SWOG myeloma trial S8229 data set. Adjusted 1% and 5% levels are shown.

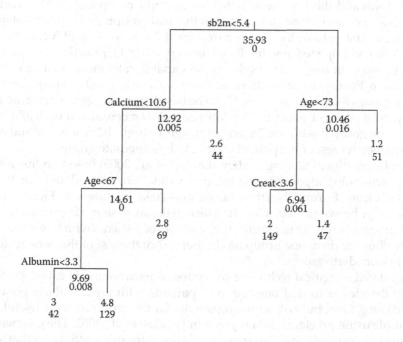

FIGURE 10.8

A regression tree based on a recursive partitioning analysis of the SWOG myeloma S8229 data set. Numbers beneath the variable names are chi-squared, adjusted *p*-value, and median.

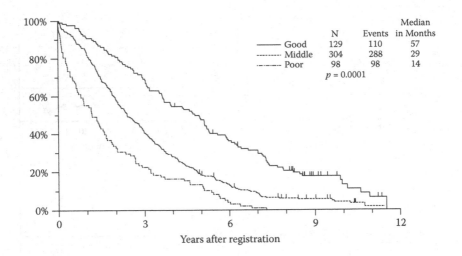

FIGURE 10.9
Prognostic groups from a recursive partitioning analysis of the SWOG myeloma trial S8229 data set.

value of the variable for each split is given, along with the logrank test statistic in χ^2 form and the *p*-value adjusted for multiple comparisons. The median survival in years and the sample size for the final groupings are also displayed. Thus the first split in the tree is based on sb2m at a value of 5.4, with a of 35.93 and an adjusted *p*-value listed as 0 ($p < 0.001$), resulting in 2 groups. The group with low sb2m is split on the variable calcium, at a value of 10.6, and so on. Finally, groups with similar survival can be combined, giving three stage groups as shown in Figure 10.9. The best prognostic group in Figure 10.9 consists of younger patients with low sb2m, low calcium and high albumin; the worst group has high sb2m and high age, or high sb2m, low age and high creatinine; the rest of the patients form the intermediate group.

An International Staging System (Greipp et al., 2005) based on this recursive partitioning algorithm and internal validation, using data from 10,000 patients from Europe, North America and Asia, is shown in Figure 10.10, which can be contrasted with the Durie-Salmon system (Figure 10.2). The best prognostic group in Figure 10.10 consists of patients with low sb2m and high albumin; the worst group has higher sb2m; the rest of the patients form the intermediate group.

A related statistical technique to recursive partitioning is called peeling. Here the idea is to find one group of patients with a particularly poor (or good) prognosis, but with enough patients for the grouping to be useful. An example using myeloma data is given in LeBlanc et al., 2002. The goal was to identify a group with median survival of 18 months or less, thinking that such a group would be a good candidate for more intensive therapy. The algorithm based on SWOG S8229 identified those with sb2m >= 10.1, constituting 17%

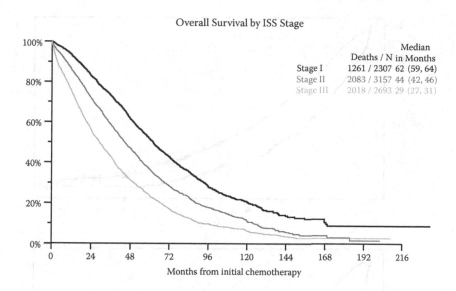

Overall Survival by ISS Stage

	Deaths / N	Median in Months
Stage I	1261 / 2307	62 (59, 64)
Stage II	2083 / 3157	44 (42, 46)
Stage III	2018 / 2693	29 (27, 31)

Months from initial chemotherapy

FIGURE 10.10
International Staging System (ISS) for myeloma, derived by recursive partitioning.

of the sample, and a second group with $10.1 > sb2m >= 4.7$, albumin < 3.7 and age $>= 68$, which added another 10%. The 2 groups together had a median survival of 18 months. In contrast, from the regression tree in Figure 10.8 one could identify those with $sb2m >= 5.4$ and age $>= 73$, along with those with $sb2m >= 5.4$, age < 73 and creatinine $>= 3.6$, constituting 19% of the sample with a median survival of 17 months. Figure 10.11 shows the results of these two approaches for finding a poor prognosis subset, applied to the data from SWOG S8229. Applying these groups to the validation data from SWOG S8624 yielded very similar survival results, with 27% of the sample in the poor prognosis group using peeling, and 15% from the regression tree approach. Note that the peeling algorithm generates a larger subset of poor prognosis patients, and so might be more useful clinically than regression trees for the purpose of isolating a single prognosis group from the rest of the patients.

10.5 Analysis of Microarray Data

The past decades have witnessed an explosion of knowledge about the human genome and the genes that play a role in the development and progression of cancer, and considerable progress in moving that knowledge from the bench to the bedside. A key to this revolution was the development of the microarray

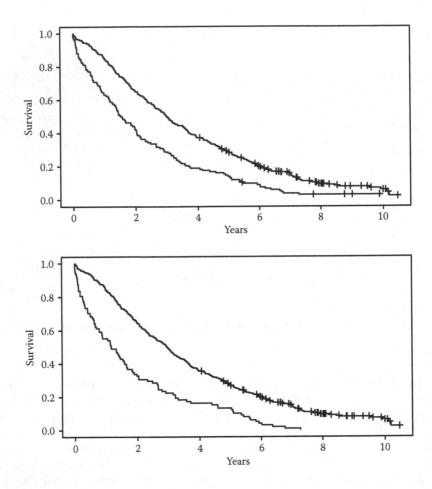

FIGURE 10.11
Survival curves for poor prognostic groups versus the remaining patients, based on data from myeloma trial S8229. The top panel is based on peeling and the bottom on regression trees.

chip, a technology which permits the researcher to study literally thousands of genes in a single assay. There are several approaches to developing these chips, but the basics are that known genes or key parts of genes (sequences of nucleotides, or probes) are fixed on a small slide, and a sample from a subject is prepared in such a way that genes that exist in the sample will attach to the genes on the slide. The output for each gene is compared to either an internal or external control and is expressed as either a categorical (gene present or not) or a measured variable (usually a ratio or a log ratio of experimental to control, quantifying the degree of over or under expression). The chips can be created to target genes hypothesized to be involved in a specific cancer (e.g., the lymphochip for studying lymphoma, Alizadeh et al., 2000) or can be quite general (one recent chip from a commercial vendor contains over 40,000 gene probes).

There are many questions that can be addressed with this new technology, among them:

- What genes or combinations of genes (what genetic profiles) differentiate normal subjects from cancer patients?
- Can genetic profiles be used to define more useful subsets of specific cancers (replacing histology or standard laboratory measurements, for example)?
- Can genetic profiles be used to develop targeted therapy against the gene products (proteins) expressed by individual patients?

If the analyses discussed in earlier sections of this chapter have been called exploratory, it should be clear that with thousands of variables on a much smaller number of patients (these chips aren't cheap), the analysis of microarray data is *highly* exploratory. Any analysis of these data is subject to extreme problems of multiple comparisons and must be confirmed on independent data sets before being given credence.

The question of differentiating normals from cancer patients, called "class prediction" by Golub et al. (1999), can be approached for each gene using familiar statistics (Rosner, 1986) such as the χ^2 (for categorical outcomes, gene on or off) or the t-test or Wilcoxon test (for measured expression ratios). To account for the fact that thousands of such statistical tests will be done, a p-value < 0.001 or less might be used instead of the usual 5% level. Regression techniques (logistic regression for categorical outcomes, simple linear regression for measured outcomes) could be used to determine if combinations of genes predict whether a sample is from the normal or the cancer "class," but the number of genes involved make this mathematically impossible. A common solution to this problem is through a data reduction technique such as principal components (Quackenbush, 2001), which replaces the original set of thousands of variables with a much smaller set (typically 10–50) of linear combinations of the original variables, chosen to capture most of the variability in the sample. Ordinary regression techniques (or neural networks, Khan et al., 2001) can then be applied to this reduced number of variables. While such techniques might predict well whether a sample is from a normal or a cancer patient and might (if validated) be used in diagnosis, the resulting regression equation is not easily interpretable (especially with neural networks).

The question of finding subsets of cancer patients based on genetic profiles, called "class discovery" by Golub et al., is much harder to address. Statistical techniques called clustering are often used in this context. Perhaps the most common such clustering algorithm is hierarchical clustering. While there are many variations, most are based on distances between gene expression ratios for patients (in 40,000 space, quite a generalization from distances in a plane, or two space!). The two closest patients are clustered together, and a

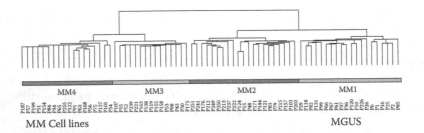

FIGURE 10.12
A dendogram from a hierarchical clustering of samples from myeloma patients, patients with MGUS, and samples from myeloma cell lines. MGUS patients clustered with the best prognosis group (MM1) and the cell lines with the worst group (MM4).

new profile is defined (by averaging or other ways) for the two-patient cluster, and the algorithm repeats until all patients are in one cluster. The result can be depicted in a tree-like structure known as a dendogram. An example using patients with multiple myeloma, as well as a few patients with a pre-myeloma condition known as monoclonal gamopathy of undetermined significance (MGUS) and a few samples from myeloma cell lines (Zhan et al., 2002), is illustrated in Figure 10.12. The investigators identified four clusters, denoted MM1-MM4, and hypothesized that these clusters represented patients with a decreasing prognosis. The fact that the MGUS patients clustered with MM1 and the cell lines (presumably from patients with advanced disease) with MM4 bolstered their conclusions. However, further follow-up for survival and independent confirmation is needed. It also should be pointed out that the hierarchical clustering algorithm always finds clusters, by definition, whether there really are important groupings or not. Other clustering routines require a prespecification of the number of clusters (usually not known, thus arbitrary) and are extremely computationally intensive (thus often requiring a preliminary data reduction step using principal components or similar methods).

Perhaps the most promising aspect of genetic profiling involves development of targeted therapy. One can foresee the day when a patient will be screened for thousands of genes and treated for the specific genetic abnormalities of his or her tumor. Cancers will be defined, staged and treated according to their genetics, not their anatomic site or appearance under a microscope. Already many agents are available which target specific gene products (from over expression of certain genes) involved in one or more cancers, including such early examples as trastuzumab (for breast cancer, lung cancer, other sites) and imatinib (for chronic myelogenous leukemia, gastrointenstinal stromal tumors, other sites), with more in the clinic and in the pipeline. Of course, the new treatments will need to be tested using the methods for clinical trials described in this book.

10.6 Meta-Analysis

The term meta-analysis seems to have been used in various ways, so at the outset let us state that we are discussing the statistical analysis of data from multiple randomized cancer clinical trials. The purposes of such meta-analyses are many, but include the testing of a null hypothesis about a given treatment in a given cancer, the estimation of the treatment effect, and the exploration of the treatment effect in subsets of patients. The fundamental reason for the growth in the interest in meta-analyses is that most cancer clinical trials are too small, so that there is little power to detect clinically meaningful differences, little precision in the estimation of such differences, and almost no value in doing subset analyses (see Chapter 9). The combination of trials into a single analysis is meant to overcome these difficulties brought about by small sample sizes for individual trials, but meta-analyses are no panacea, as we shall see.

10.6.1 Some Principles of Meta-Analyses

As with any statistical analysis, a meta-analysis can be done well or done poorly. Too often results from an arbitrary selection of tangentially related published results are thrown together and termed a meta-analysis. Conclusions from such poorly done analyses are clinically uninterpretable. Principles for a valid meta-analysis include the following:

- All trials must be included, published or not. Identification of all such trials may be the most difficult part of a meta-analysis. Including only those trials that have been published runs the risk of the well-known bias toward the publication of positive trials.

- The raw data from each trial must be retrieved and reanalyzed. This allows a common endpoint to be estimated, with standard errors, from each trial. Published data are almost never sufficient for this purpose since different studies will have used different endpoint definitions and will have presented different endpoints in the results sections of manuscripts. Use of the raw data gives the opportunity to employ a uniform set of inclusion criteria and to update the survival results, which besides resulting in more mature data also reduces the bias resulting from trials that stopped early in one-sided monitoring situations (Green et al., 1987).

- One must be wary of lumping fundamentally different interventions into one meta-analysis. Treatment regimens often differ in fundamental ways that could affect efficacy, such as dose, dose intensity, dose modifying agents, or route and timing of administration. Truly disparate interventions should not be forced into a single measure of treatment benefit. Each trial should be presented in summary form and the overall analysis (if any!) should be done by stratifying on the trials, not by collapsing over trials.

- Some measure of the quality of the trials should be incorporated into the analysis. Sensitivity analyses using different weights for each trial (including leaving some trials out altogether) should be performed.

10.6.2 An Example Meta-Analysis: Portal Vein Infusion

We will discuss several aspects of meta-analysis in the context of a specific example concerning the value of portal vein infusion of 5-fluorouracil after surgery for colorectal cancer. A more detailed exposition can be found in Crowley et al. (1994). The liver is a frequent site of failure after resection in colorectal cancer patients, and metastases reach the liver via the portal vein. Thus Taylor and colleagues at the University of Liverpool performed a randomized trial of perioperative portal vein infusion of 5-FU versus surgery alone for the treatment of non-metastatic colorectal cancer (Taylor et al., 1979; Taylor et al., 1985). The experimental arm consisted of the infusion of one gram of 5-FU daily by catheter into the portal vein for the first seven postoperative days (heparin was also given to prevent thrombosis). Eligible patients included those with Dukes' A, B, or C colorectal cancer. The result was a dramatic difference in favor of 5-FU infusion via the portal vein versus controls, both in survival and in the incidence of hepatic metastases as a site of first failure. There was a 50% reduction in the hazard rate for the experimental group and a 4% incidence of liver metastases against 17% in the control group, but with a total sample size of less than 250 "evaluable" patients for this adjuvant trial, the confidence limits were rather wide, and the authors wisely called for confirmatory trials.

Since then nine such confirmatory trials have been completed. The results of these trials can best be described as mixed; some show an effect on liver metastases but little or no effect on survival, some show a survival benefit but no difference in liver metastases, some show neither, and some claim to show both. The largest trial was performed by the NSABP (Wolmark et al., 1990; Wolmark et al., 1993). Approximately 750 eligible patients were randomized to the same two arms as in the Liverpool trial, with small survival differences emerging at about 30 months but no differences in the incidence of liver metastases. The authors attribute any treatment effect to a systemic one, not one localized to the liver. In an attempt to sort out the issues, a formal meta-analysis has been performed by the Liver Infusion Meta-Analysis Group (1997). We review the issues faced by the authors of this effort, as a way to illustrate the promise and problems of meta-analyses.

10.6.2.1 Inclusion of Trials

A great deal of effort went into identifying trials for the portal vein infusion meta-analysis, as attested by the inclusion of a trial presented only in abstract form. But are there trials (most likely negative) that haven't even been presented in abstract form? While inclusion of all trials is the best way to avoid publication bias, it does increase the likelihood that trials of highly variable quality will be assembled for analysis. A related issue is whether the initial trial should be included in the meta-analysis, since in cases such as this one where a positive trial is the catalyst for confirmatory trials, the first study almost certainly overestimates the treatment benefit. The Liver Infusion Meta-Analysis Group (LIMG) addressed this issue by providing analyses both including and excluding the Taylor trial.

10.6.2.2 Use of Raw Data

The LIMG gathered raw data from each investigator. This allowed them to define relative risk as a common measure of treatment benefit and to calculate standard errors of the estimate from each trial. The incidence of liver metastases is subject to the problem of competing risks (see Chapter 9), however, and having the raw data does not solve that problem. Some of the heterogeneity in eligibility criteria in these trials (e.g., the inclusion of Dukes' A patients or not) can be handled (through stratified analyses) only if the raw data are analyzed. Several of the trials excluded treatment violations from their reports, but the intent-to-treat analysis was restored in the meta-analysis. In fact, all patients, eligible or not, were included, apparently in the belief that it is better to guard against the possible biases introduced by inappropriate or selective enforcement of eligibility criteria than to restrict the variability by excluding patients not likely to benefit from treatment.

10.6.2.3 Lumping Interventions

All of the trials delivered 5-FU via the portal vein for one week, starting with surgery. There were variations in the dose of 5-FU, but most would probably regard these as minor. Thus the trials included in the meta-analysis can be argued to be testing a comparable intervention. This is in stark contrast to many of the other such efforts we have been involved with. A recent literature-based meta-analysis we reviewed compared single agent versus combination chemotherapy in advanced non-small cell lung cancer, without regard to which single agent, which combination, or which doses. Other recent examples address the value of "chemotherapy" in head and neck cancer without regard to which agents, and the possible benefit of "radiotherapy" in limited small-cell lung cancer, without regard to timing (concomitant or sequential), dose, or fractionation. It is doubtful whether any formal analysis of existing trials can sort out such complex issues.

10.6.2.4 Quality of Trials

Our own review of the portal-vein infusion trials revealed considerable heterogeneity with respect to their quality. Some of the deficiencies can be rectified in a meta-analysis of the raw data, some cannot. The sample size was inadequate for all but extremely unrealistic differences in all but one of the trials and most were reported too early (a few had no follow-up data on some patients at the time of publication). While meta-analysis does result in larger numbers and can present updated survival data, in at least one trial no such updates were possible (the trial organization having terminated).

The most serious problems with the individual studies involved the timing of randomization and exclusions from analysis. As stated in Chapter 6, randomization should take place as close in time as possible to the point where treatments first diverge. In trials of portal vein infusion via catheter placed at surgery, there is the option of randomizing preoperatively or intraoperatively. Preoperative randomization was done in about half of the trials, and resulted in from 2% to 38% of patients declared ineligible at surgery (because of metastatic disease not detected before surgery, or an inability to perform a curative resection, for example). There is the possibility that a retrospective review of such cases for ineligibility could be biased due to knowledge of the treatment assignment. Intraoperative randomization in the other trials resulted in ineligibility rates (largely for reasons known in principle before randomization) that ranged from 2% to 14%. While all ineligibles were included in the meta-analysis, eliminating such biases, one still wonders about the overall quality of some of the studies, and whether the ineligible patients were followed with the same rigor as the eligible ones.

Taylor reported the exclusion from the analysis of 7% of patients in whom a catheter could not be placed, which destroys the balance created at randomization and introduces biases in the analysis. Only patients randomized to portal vein infusion have the chance to be excluded as protocol violations, and they could well have a different prognosis from the remainder of patients. In other trials this was either not done or happened in only a few cases. Again, the meta-analysis using all the data can in theory rectify such problems, but Taylor reported that the patients excluded due to protocol violations were lost to follow-up.

10.6.3 Conclusions from the Portal Vein Meta-Analysis

The LIMG concluded from their meta-analysis that there was a benefit for portal vein infusion over observation (relative risk $= 0.86$, $p = 0.006$) but noted that the strength of that conclusion depended heavily on whether or not the original trial of Taylor was included in the meta-analysis. They called for more randomized evidence. Our conclusion from a more informal review of the individual trials is that the usefulness of this approach is unproven. Combining nine trials of uneven quality did not result in one good trial. The only trial of adequate size demonstrated a very small, late-appearing improvement in survival, and no effect on liver metastases. Since adjuvant therapy with 5-FU and levamisole starting 1 month after surgery has been shown to be of benefit over observation at least for Dukes' C patients (Moertel et al., 1990), our review suggests that the relevant question is not about infusion but whether early systemic therapy, beginning right after surgery, adds benefit to conventional adjuvant therapy. This was tested in an intergroup trial coordinated by the Eastern Cooperative Oncology Group, INT-0136, with results still pending. The controversy continues (Biagi et al., 2011).

10.6.4 Some Final Remarks on Meta-Analysis

Our inclusion of this topic in a chapter on exploratory analyses is an indication of our belief that the importance of meta-analyses lies mainly in exploration, not confirmation. In settling therapeutic issues, a meta-analysis is a poor substitute for one large, well-conducted trial. In particular, the expectation that a meta-analysis will be done does not justify designing studies that are too small to detect realistic differences with adequate power. Done well, a meta-analysis is a good review of existing data, and can provide an idea of the plausible magnitude of treatment benefit and generate hypotheses about treatment effects in subsets. However, there is a tendency to view the results of meta-analyses as being more definitive than they really are (Machtay et al., 1999). As pointed out by Kassirer (1992), there is a near certainty that the studies collected for a meta-analysis are heterogeneous in their designs, and thus shouldn't be thought of as providing estimates of a single quantity. The statistical techniques for accounting for this variability are controversial (see Marubini and Valsecchi, 1995, for a discussion). The quality of each trial needs to be taken into account, at least informally. With a very large meta-analysis, one also needs to keep in mind that not all statistically significant results are clinically meaningful.

10.7 Concluding Remarks

One approach to cancer clinical trials, espoused by Richard Peto (Peto et al., 1976), is for the "large, simple trial." There is much to commend this attitude, and we are sympathetic with the goal of designing clinical trials that are large enough to yield definitive answers to important clinical questions. Each secondary objective with its associated additional data requirements jeopardizes the ability to answer the primary question, and eventually the trial submerges of its own weight. Yet, one does want to learn something even from negative trials, so the urge to add limited secondary objectives is almost irresistible. We have tried to illustrate here, in the context of exploratory analyses using survival data, what might be learned from a trial or sequence of trials beyond answers to the primary treatment questions, and what the limitations are of such explorations. Further, we have tried to indicate that performing one large trial well is much to be preferred over combining several smaller ones.

11

Summary and Conclusions

- The grand thing is to be able to reason backwards.
- There is nothing more deceptive than an obvious fact.
- The temptation to form premature theories upon insufficient data is the bane of our profession.
- It is an error to argue in front of your data. You find yourself insensibly twisting them round to fit your theories.

—**Sherlock Holmes**

Sherlock Holmes had it right. Reasoning backward from data to truth is full of traps and pitfalls. Statistics helps us to avoid the traps and to reason correctly. The main points we have tried to make in this book about such reasoning can be summarized briefly as follows:

- Clinical research searches for answers in an heterogeneous environment. Large variability, little understood historical trends, and unquantifiable but undoubtedly large physician and patient biases for one or another treatment are all indications for carefully controlled, randomized clinical trials.
- Statistical principles (and thus statisticians) have a large role (but certainly not the only role) in the design, conduct, and analysis of clinical trials.
- Careful attention to design is essential for the success of such trials. Agreement needs to be reached among all parties as to the objectives, endpoints and definitions thereof, population to be studied and thus the eligibility criteria for the trial, treatments to be studied, and potential benefits of treatment to be detected with what limits of precision or statistical error probabilities (defining sample size).
- Two-arm trials have the virtue of a high likelihood of being able to answer one question well. Multi-arm trials should only be conducted with adequate sample size to protect against multiple comparisons and multiple other problems, and should not be based on untested and unlikely assumptions regarding how treatments will behave in combinations.

- The analysis of trials as they unfold should be presented only to a select, knowledgeable few who are empowered to make decisions, using statistical guidelines, as to whether the results are so convincing that accrual should be stopped, that the trial should be reported early, or that other fundamental changes should be made.

- Careful attention to the details of data quality, including clear and concise protocols, data definitions, forms and protocols; quality control and quality assurance measures; and database management is crucial to the success of trials.

- All completed trials should be reported in the literature, with a thorough accounting of all patients entered and a clear statistical analysis of all eligible patients on the arm to which they were assigned.

- There is no substitute for a randomized trial of adequate sample size with clinical endpoints for answering questions about the benefit of cancer treatments. Historical controls are completely unreliable, retrospective analyses of groups defined by their response or their attained dose are subject to irreparable biases, and the use of short-term endpoints of little clinical relevance can lead to seriously flawed conclusions.

- The protocol-stated analysis of the primary endpoint should result in an unassailable conclusion of a clinical trial. Any other analyses are secondary. The data should be explored to generate hypotheses for future research; this is a familiar province of the statistician, but be aware that there is more art (and thus less reproducibility) than science in this endeavor. Meta-analyses should be viewed as exploratory, and as supplements to but not as substitutes for large randomized trials.

- Clinical trials are a complex undertaking and a fragile enterprise. Every complication, every extra data item, every extra arm should be viewed with the suspicion that their addition might jeopardize the whole trial. Make sure one important question is answered well, then see what else might be learned.

Recently we were asked to write a mission statement for the SWOG Statistical Center. Here is our view:

> The primary mission of the Southwest Oncology Group Statistical Center is to make progress in the prevention and cure of cancer through clinical research. The mission is accomplished through the conduct of important trials and through translation of biologic concepts. Quality research, quality data and publication of results are critical to the effort. The statistical center contributes through:
>
> Study Design. The statistical center has a fundamental role in clarifying study objectives and in designing statistically sound studies to meet those objectives.

Protocol Review. The statistical center reviews all protocols for logical consistency and completeness, in order that study conduct not be compromised through use of an inaccurate protocol document.

Data Quality Control and Study Monitoring. The statistical center continually enters, forwards to study coordinators, reviews, corrects, updates, and stores data from all active Southwest Oncology Group studies, in order that study results not be compromised by flawed data and that studies be monitored for patient safety.

Analysis and Publication. The statistical center is responsible for statistical analysis and interpretation of all Southwest Oncology Group coordinated studies and all Southwest Oncology Group database studies.

Statistical Research. The statistical center has an active research program addressing unresolved design and analysis issues important to the conduct of cancer clinical trials and to ancillary biologic studies.

We hope that this book has contributed to an understanding of how we conduct ourselves in fulfillment of this mission.

References

Aickin M. Randomization, balance, and the validity and efficiency of design-adaptive allocation methods. *Journal of Statistical Planning and Inference* 94:97–119, 2001.

Alberts D. S., Green S., Hannigan E. V., O'Toole R., Stock-Novak D., Anderson P., Surwit E. A., Malviya V. K., Nahhas W. A., and Jolles C. J. Improved therapeutic index of carboplatin plus cyclophosphamide versus cisplatin plus cyclophosphamide: Final report by the Southwest Oncology Group of a phase III randomized trial in stages III and IV ovarian cancer. *Journal of Clinical Oncology* 10:706–717, 1992.

Alizadeh A. A., Eisen M. B., Davis R. E., Ma C., Lossos I. S., Rosenwald A., Boldrick J. C., Sabet H., Tran T., Yu X., Powell J. I., Yand L., Marti G. E., Moore T., Hudson J. Jr., Lu L., Lewis D. B., Tibshirani R., Sherlock G., Chan W. C., Greiner T. C., Weisenburger D. D., Armitage J. O., Warnke R., Levy R., Wilson W., Grever M. R., Byrd J. C., Botstein D., Brown P. O., and Staudt L. M. Distinct types of diffuse large B-cell lymphoma identified by gene expression profiling. *Nature* 403:503–511, 2000.

Altaman L. US Halts Recruitment of Cancer Patients for Studies, Pointing to Flaws in Oversight. *New York Times*, Wed. March 30, p A-12, 1994.

Anderson J. R., Cain K. C., and Gelber R. D. Analysis of survival by tumor response. *Journal of Clinical Oncology* 1:710–719, 1983.

Anderson P. K. Conditional power calculations as an aid in the decision whether to continue a clinical trial. *Controlled Clinical Trials* 8:67–74, 1987.

Anderson G. L., LeBlanc M., Liu P. Y., and Crowley J. On use of covariates in randomization and analysis of clinical trials. In *Handbook of Statistics in Clinical Oncology*, 2nd edition. J. Crowley and D. P. Ankerst (eds.). Boca Raton, FL: Chapman and Hall/CRC Press, pp 167–180, 2006.

Antman K., Crowley J., Balcerzak S. P., Rivkin S. E., Weiss G. R., Elias A., Natale R. B., et al. An intergroup phase III randomized study of doxorubicin and dacarbazine with or without ifosfamide and mesna in advanced soft tissue and bone sarcomas. *Journal of Clinical Oncology* 11:1276–1285, 1993.

Babb J., Rogatko A., and Zacks S. Cancer phase I clinical trials: Efficient dose escalation with overdose control. *Statistics in Medicine* 17:1103–1120, 1998.

Balcerzak S., Benedetti J., Weiss G. R., and Natale R. B. A phase II trial of paclitaxel in patients with advanced soft tissue sarcomas: A Southwest Oncology Group study. *Cancer* 76:2248–2252, 1995.

Barlogie B., Anderson K., Berenson J., Crowley J., Cunningham D., Gertz M., Henon P., et al. In K. Dicke and A. Keeting (eds.): *Autologous Marrow and Blood Transplantation. Proceedings of the Seventh International Symposium.* Arlington, TX. pp 399–410, 1995.

Barlogie B., Kyle R., Anderson K., Greipp P., Lazarus H., Hurd D., McCoy J., et al. Standard chemotherapy compared with high-dose chemoradiotherapy for multiple myeloma: Final results of phase III US intergroup trial S9321. *Journal of Clinical Oncology* 24:929–935, 2006.

Bartlett R., Roloff D., Cornell R., Andrews A., Dillon P., and Zwischenberger J. Extracorporeal circulation in neonatal respiratory failure: A prospective randomized study. *Pediatrics* 76:476–487, 1985.

Battaille R., Durie B. G. M., and Grenier J. Serum beta-2 microglobulin and survival duration in multiple myeloma: A simple reliable marker for staging. *British Journal of Haematology* 55:439–447, 1983.

Bauer P. and Kieser M. Combining different phase in the development of medical treatments within a single trial. *Statistics in Medicine* 18:1833–1848, 1999.

Begg C. B. and Kalish L. A. Treatment allocation for nonlinear models in clinical trials: The logistic model. *Biometrics* 40:409–420, 1984.

Bekele B. and Shen Y. A Bayesian approach to jointly modeling toxicity and biomarker expression in a Phase I/II dose-finding trial. *Biometrics* 61:344–354, 2005.

Benedetti J. K., Liu P.-Y., Sather H., Seinfeld H., and Epson M. Effective sample size for censored survival data. *Biometrika* 69:343–349, 1982.

Berlin J., Stewart J. A., Storer B., Tutsch K. D., Arzoomanin R. Z., Alberti D., Feierabend C., Simon K., and Wilding G. Phase I clinical and pharmacokinetic trial of penclomedine using a novel, two-stage trial design for patients with advanced malignancy. *Journal of Clinical Oncology* 16:1142–1149, 1998.

Bernard C. L. *Introduction à l'Etude de la Médecine Expérimentale*. 1866, reprinted, Garnier-Flammarion, London 1966.

Bernstein D. and Lagakos S. Sample size and power determination for stratified clinical trials. *Journal of Statistical Computations and Simulation* 8:65–73, 1978.

Berry D. A. Adaptive clinical trials: The promise and the caution. *Journal of Clinical Oncology* 29:606–609, 2011.

Biagi J. J., Raphael M. J., Mackillop W. J., Kong W., King W. D., and Booth C. M. Association between time to initiation of adjuvant chemotherapy and survival in colorectal cancer: A systematic review and meta-analysis. *Journal of the American Medical Association* 305:2335–2342, 2011.

Blackwelder W. C. "Proving the null hypothesis" in clinical trials. *Controlled Clinical Trials* 3:345–353, 1982.

Blumenstein B. A. The relational database model and multiple multicenter clinical trials. *Controlled Clinical Trials* 10:386–406, 1989.

Boissel J.-P. Impact of randomized clinical trials on medical practices. *Controlled Clinical Trials* 10:120S–134S, 1989.

Bonadonna G. and Valagussa P. Dose-response effect of adjuvant chemotherapy in breast cancer. *New England Journal of Medicine* 34:10–15, 1981.

Boutron I., Estellat C., and Ravaud P. A review of blinding in randomized controlled trials found results inconsistent and questionable. *Journal of Clinical Epidemiology* 58:1220–1226, 2005.

Breiman L., Friedman J. H., Olshen R. A., and Stone C. J. *Classification and Regression Trees*. Belmont, CA: Wadsworth International Group, 1984.

Breslow N. and Crowley J. Large sample properties of the life table and PL estimates under random censorship. *Annals of Statistics* 2:437–453, 1972.

Brookmeyer R. and Crowley J. A confidence interval for the median survival time. *Biometrics* 38:29–41, 1982.

Bryant J. and Day R. Incorporating toxicity considerations into the design of two-stage phase II clinical trials. *Biometrics* 51:1372–1383, 1995.

Budd G. T., Green S., O'Bryan R. M., Martino S., Abeloff M. D., Rinehart J. J., Hahn R., et al. Short-course FAC-M versus 1 year of CMFVP in node-positive, hormone receptor-negative breast cancer: An intergroup study. *Journal of Clinical Oncology* 13:831–839, 1995.

Bunn P. A., Crowley J., Kelly K., Hazuka M. B., Beasley K., Upchurch C., and Livingston R. Chemoradiotherapy with or without granulocyte-macrophage colony-stimulating factor in the treatment of limited-stage small-cell lung cancer: A prospective Phase III randomized study of the Southwest Oncology Group. *Journal of Clinical Oncology* 13:1632–1641, 1995.

Burkhardt B., Woessmann W., Zimmermann M., Kontny U., Vormoor J., Doerffel W., Mann G., et al. Impact of cranial radiotherapy on central nervous system prophylaxis in children and adolescents with central nervous system—negative Stage III or IV lymphoblastic lymphoma. *Journal of Clinical Oncology* 24:491–499, 2006.

Burris H. A., Moore M. J., Andersen J., Green M. R., Rothenberg M. L., Modiano M. R., Cripps M. C., et al. Improvements in survival and clinical benefit with gemcitabine as first-line therapy for patients with advanced pancreas cancer; a randomized trial. *Journal of Clinical Oncology* 15:2403–2417, 1997.

Buyse M. and Molenberghs G. Criteria for the validation of surrogate endpoints in randomized experiments. *Biometrics* 54:1014–1029, 1998.

Byar D. P., Simon R. M., Friedewalde W. T., Schlesselman J. J., DeMets D. L., Ellenberg J. H., Gail M. H., and Ware J. H. Randomized clinical trials: Perspectives on some recent ideas. *New England Journal of Medicine* 295:74–80, 1976.

Chang M., Therneau T., Wieand H. S., and Cha S. Designs for group sequential Phase II clinical trials. *Biometrics* 43:865–874, 1987.

Chang M. N. and O'Brien P. C. Confidence intervals following group seqential tests. *Controlled Clinical Trials* 7:18–26, 1986.

Chang M., Devidas M., and Anderson J. One- and two-stage designs for phase II window studies. *Statistics in Medicine* 26:2604–2614, 2007.

Chen T. and Simon R. Extension of one-sided test to multiple treatment trials. *Controlled Clinical Trials* 15:124–134, 1994.

Cheung C., Liu Y., Wong K., Chan H., Chan Y., Wong H., Chak W., et al. Can daclizumab reduce acute rejection and improve long-term renal function in tacrolimus-based primary renal transplant recipients? *Nephrology* 13:251–255, 2008.

Christian M. C., McCabe M. S., Korn E. L., Abrams J. S., Kaplan R. S., and Friedman M. A. The National Cancer Institute audit of the National Surgical Adjuvant Breast and Bowel Project Protocol B-06. *New England Journal of Medicine* 333:1469–1474, 1995.

Chu P.-L., Lin Y., and Shih W. J. Unifying CRM and EWOC designs for phase I cancer clinical trials. *Journal of Statistical Planning and Inference* 139:1146–1163, 2009.

Ciampi A., Thiffault J., Nakache J.-P., and Asselain B. Stratification by stepwise regression, correspondence analysis and recursive partitioning. *Computatutional Statistics and Data Analysis* 4:185–204, 1986.

Clark D. A., Stinson E. B., Griepp R. B., Schroeder J. S., Shumway N. E., and Harrison D. C. Cardiac transplantation in man, VI. Prognosis of patients selected for cardia transplantation. *Annals of Internal Medicine* 75:15–21, 1971.

Cobo M., Isla D., Massuti B., Montes A., Sanchez J. M., Provencio M., Viñolas N., et al. Customizing cisplatin based on quantitative excision repair cross-complementing 1 mRNA expression: A phase III trial in non–small-cell lung cancer. *Journal of Clinical Oncology* 25:2747–2754, 2007.

Collins J. M., Zaharko D. S., Dedrick R. L., and Chabner B. A. Potential roles for preclinical pharmacology in Phase I clinical trials. *Cancer Treatment Reports* 70:73–80, 1986.

Collins J. M., Grieshaber C. K., and Chabner B. A. Pharmacologically guided Phase I clinical trials based upon preclinical drug development. *Journal of the National Cancer Institute* 82:1321–1326, 1990.

Collins J. M. Innovations in Phase I design: Where do we go next? *Clinical Cancer Research* 6:3801–3802, 2000.

Collins R. and MacMahon S. Reliable assessment of the effects of treatment on mortality and major morbidity, I: Clinical trials. *Lancet* 357: 373–380, 2001.

Conaway M. R. and Petroni G. R. Bivariate sequential designs for phase II trials. *Biometrics* 51:656–664, 1995.

Concorde Coordinating Committee. Concorde: MRC/ANRS randomized double-blind controlled trial of immediate and deferred zidovudine in symtom-free HIV infection. *Lancet* 343:871–881, 1994.

Cook R. J. and Farewell V. T. Guidelines for monitoring efficacy and toxicity response in clinical trials. *Biometrics* 50:1146–1152, 1994.

Cooper R., Holland J., and Glidewell O. Adjuvant chemotherapy of breast cancer. *Cancer* 44:793–798, 1979.

Coronary Drug Project Research Group. Influence of adherence to treatment and response of cholesterol on mortality in the coronary drug project. *New England Journal of Medicine* 303:1038–1041, 1980.

Cowan J. D., Green S., Neidhart J., McClure S., Coltman C. Jr., Gumbart C., Martino S., et al. Randomized trial of doxorubicin, bisantrene and mitoxantrone in advanced breast cancer. A Southwest Oncology Group study. *Journal of the National Cancer Institute* 83:1077–1084, 1991.

Cox D. R. Regression models and life-tables (with discussion). *Journal of the Royal Statistical Society, Series B* 34:187–220, 1972.

Crowley J. and Breslow N. Statistical analysis of survival data. *Annual Review of Public Health* 5:385–411, 1984.

Crowley J. Perioperative portal vein chemotherapy. In *ASCO Educational Book*, 30th Annual Meeting, Dallas, TX, 1994.

Crowley J., Green S., Liu P.-Y., and Wolf M. Data monitoring committees and early stopping guidelines: The Southwest Oncology Group experience. *Statistics in Medicine* 13:1391–1399, 1994.

Crowley J., LeBlanc M., Gentleman R., and Salmon S. Exploratory methods in survival analysis. In H. L. Koul and J. V. Deshpande, Eds. *Analysis of Censored Data*. Hayward, CA: IMS Lecture Notes-Monograph Series 27:55–77, 1995.

Crowley J., LeBlanc M., Jacobson J., and Salmon S. E. Some exploratory methods for survival data. In D.-Y. Lin and T. R. Fleming, Eds. *Proceedings of the First Seattle Symposium on Biostatistics*. Springer-Verlag, 1997.

De Moulin, D. *A Short History of Breast Cancer*. Dordrecht Germany: Kluwer Academic, 1989.

DeMets D. L., Fleming T. R., Whitley R., Childress J. F., Ellenberg S. S., Foulkes M., Mayer K. H., et al. The data and safety monitoring board and acquired immune deficiency syndrome (AIDS) trials. *Controlled Clinical Trials* 16:408–421, 1995.

Dees E. C., Whitfield L. R., Grove W. R., Rummel S., Grochow L. B., and Donehower R. C. A phase I and pharmacologic evaluation of the DNA intercalator CI-958 in patients with advanced solid tumors. *Clinical Cancer Research* 6:3801–3802, 2000.

Diem K. and Lentner C. (eds.). *Scientific Tables*. Basel, Switzerland: J. R. Geigy, 1970.

Dimond E. G., Kittle C. F., and Crockett J. E. Comparison of internal mammary artery ligation and sham operation for angina pectoris. *American Journal of Cardiology* 5:483–486, 1960.

Dixon D. and Simon R. Sample size consideration for studies comparing survival curves using historical controls. *Journal of Clinical Epidemiology* 41:1209–1213, 1988.

Dmitrienko A., Tamhane A., Bretz F. (eds.). *Multiple Testing Problems in Pharmaceutical Statistics.* Boca Raton, FL: Chapman and Hall/CRC, 2009.

Dodd L. E., Korn E. L., Friedlin B., Jaffee C. C., Rubenstein L. V., Dancey J., and Mooney M. M. Blinded independent central review of progression-free survival in phase III oncology trials: Important design element or unnecessary expense? *Journal of Clinical Oncology* 26:3791–3796, 2008.

Draper N. R. and Smith H. *Applied Regression Analysis.* New York: Wiley, 1968.

Duffy D. E. and Santner T. J. Confidence intervals for a binomial parameter based on multistage tests. *Biometrics* 43:81–94, 1987.

Durie B. G. M. and Salmon S. E. A clinical system for multiple myeloma. Correlation of measured myeloma cell mass with presenting clinical features, response to treatment and survival. *Cancer* 36:842–854, 1975.

Durie B. G. M., Dixon D. O., Carter S., Stephens R., Rivkin S., Bonnet J., Salmon S. E., Dabich L., Files J. C., and Costanzi J. Improved survival duration with combination induction for multiple myeloma: A Southwest Oncology Group study. *Journal of Clinical Oncology* 4:1227–1237, 1986.

Duvillard E. E. *Analyse et tableaux de l'influence de la petite vérole sur la mortalité à chaque âge, et de celle qu'un préservatif tel que la vaccine peut avoir sur la population et la longevité.* Paris: Imprimerie Imperiale, 1806.

Echt D. S., Liebson P. R., Mitchell L. B. et al. Mortality and morbidity in patients receiveing ecainide, flecainide or placebo: The Cardiac Arrythmia Suppression Trial. *New England Journal of Medicine* 324:781–788, 1991.

Ederer F. Jerome Cornfield's contributions to the conduct of clinical trials. *Biometrics (Supplement)* 38:25–32, 1982.

Edge S. B., Byrd D. R., Compton C. C., Fritz A. G., Greene F. L., and Trotti A. (eds.). *AJCC Cancer Staging Manual,* 7th ed. New York: Springer, 2010.

Eisenhauer E. A., O'Dwyer P. J., Christian M., and Humphrey J. S. Phase I clinical trial design in cancer drug development. *Journal of Clinical Oncology* 18:684–692, 2000.

Eisenhauer E. A., Therasse P., Bogaert J., Schwartz L. H., Sargent D., Ford R., Dancey J., et al. New response evaluation criteria in solid tumours: Revised RECIST guideline (version 1.1). *European Journal of Cancer* 45:228–247, 2009.

Ellenberg S. Randomization designs in comparative clinical trials. *New England Journal of Medicine* 310:1404–1408, 1984.

Ellenberg S. S., Finkelstein D. M., and Schoenfeld D. A. Statistical issues arising in AIDS clinical trials. *Journal of the American Statistical Association* 87:562–569, 1992.

Faraggi D., LeBlanc M., and Crowley J. Understanding neural networks using regression trees: An application to multiple myeloma survival data. *Statistics in Medicine* 20:2965–2976, 2001.

Fisher B. Winds of change in clinical trials—from Daniel to Charlie Brown. *Controlled Clinical Trials* 4:65–74, 1983.

Fisher R., Gaynor E., Dahlberg S., Oken M., Grogan T., Mize E., Glick J., Coltman C., and Miller T. Comparison of a standard regimen (CHOP) with three intensive chemotherapy regimens for advanced non-Hodgkin's lymphoma. *New England Journal of Medicine* 328:1002–1006, 1993.

Fleiss J. L. *Statistical Methods for Rates and Proportions*, 2nd ed. New York: Wiley, 1981.

Fleiss J. L., Tytun A., and Ury H. K. A simple approximation for calculating sample sizes for comparing independent proportions. *Biometrics* 36:343–346, 1980.

Fleming T. One sample multiple testing procedures for Phase II clinical trials. *Biometrics* 38:143–151, 1982.

Fleming T. R. Evaluating therapeutic interventions: Some issues and experiences. *Statistical Science* 7:428–456, 1992.

Fleming T., Green S., and Harrington P. Considerations for monitoring and evaluating treatment effects in clinical trials. *Controlled Clinical Trials* 5:55–66, 1984.

Fleming T. R. Interpretation of subgroup analyses in clinical trials. *Drug Information Journal* 29:1681S–1687S, 1995.

Food and Drug Administration. Guidance for Industry: E10. Choice of control group and related issues in clinical trials. Office of Training and Communication. *Center for Drug Evaluation and Research*. Rockville MD, 2001.

Food and Drug Administration Guidance for Industry: Noninferiority clinical trials. Draft, 2010.

Freeman T., Vawtner D., Leaverton P., Godbold J., Hauser R., Goetz C., and Olanow C. W. Use of placebo surgery in controlled trials of a cellular based therapy for Parkinson's disease. *New England Journal of Medicine* 341:988–992, 1999.

Frei E. III, Holland J. F., Schneiderman M. A., Pinkel D., Selkirk C., Freireich E. J., Silver R. T., Gold C. L., and Regelson W. A comparative study of two regimens of combination chemotherapy in acute leukemia. *Blood* 13:1126–1148, 1958.

Frytak S., Moertel C., O'Fallon J., Rubin J., Creagan E., O'Connel M., Schutt A., and Schwartau N. Delta-9-Tetrahydrocannabinol as an antiemetic for patients receiving cancer chemotherapy. *Annals of Internal Medicine* 91:825–830, 1979.

Gail M. H. Statistics in action. *Journal of the American Statistical Association* 91:1–13, 1996.

Gallo P., Chuang-Stein C., Dragalin V., Gaydos B., Krams M., and Pinheiro J. Adaptive designs in clinical drug development—and executive summary of the PhRMA working group. *Journal of Biopharmaceutical Statistics* 16:275–283, 2006.

Gandara D. R., Crowley J., Livingston R. B., Perez E. A., Taylor C. W., Weiss G., Neefe J. R., et al. Evaluation of cisplatin in metastatic non-small cell lung cancer: A phase III study of the Southwest Oncology Group. *Journal of Clinical Oncology* 11:873–878, 1993.

Gehan E. A generalized Wilcoxon test for comparing arbitrarily singly-censored samples. *Biometrika* 52:203–223, 1965.

Gelmon K., Latreille J., Tolcher A., Génier L., Fisher B., Forand D., D'Aloisio S., et al. Phase I dose-finding study of a new taxane, RPR 109881A, administered as a one-hour intravenous infusion days 1 and 8 to patients with advanced solid tumors. *Journal of Clinical Oncology* 18:4098–108, 2000.

Gentleman R. and Crowley J. Local full likelihood estimation for the proportional hazards model. *Biometrics* 47:1283–1296, 1991a.

Gentleman R. and Crowley J. Graphical methods for censored data. *Journal of the American Statistical Association* 86:678–682, 1991b.

George S. A survey of monitoring practices in cancer clinical trials. *Statistics in Medicine* 12:435–450, 1993.

Gil Deza E., Balbiani L., Coppola F., Blajman C., Block J. F., Giachella O., Chacon R., Capo A., Zori Comba A., Fein L., Polera L., Matwiejuk M., Jaremtchuk A., Muro H., Reale M., Bass C., Chiesa G., Van Koten M., and Schmilovich A. Phase III study of navelbine (NVB) vs NVB plus cisplatin in non small cell lung cancer (NSCLC) Stage IIIB or IV. *Proceedings of ASCO* 15:39 (#1193), 1996.

Gilbert J. P., McPeek B., and Mosteller F. Statistics and ethics in surgery and anesthesia. *Science* 198:684–689, 1977.

Gold P. J., Goldman B., Iqbal S., Leichman L. P., Zhang W., Lenz H. J., and Blanke C. D. Cetuximab as second-line therapy in patients with metastatic esophageal adenocarcinoma: A phase II Southwest Oncology Group Study (S0415). *Journal of Thoracic Oncology* 5:1472–1476, 2010.

Goldberg K. B. and Goldberg P. (eds.). *Four Patients in Tamoxifen Treatment Trial Had Died of Uterine Cancer Prior to BCPT. The Cancer Letter*, April 29, 1994.

Goldie J. H., Coldman A. J., and Gudauskas G. A. Rationale for the use of alternating non-cross-resistant chemotherapy. *Cancer Treatment Reports* 66:439–449, 1982.

Goldman B., LeBlanc M., and Crowley J. Interim futility analysis with intermediate endpoints. *Clinical Trials* 5:14–22, 2008.

Golub T. R., Slonim D. K., Tamoyo P., Huard C., Gaasenbeck M., Mesiriv J. P., Coller H., Loh M. L., Dowving J. R., Caliguri M. A., Bloomfield C. D., and Lander E. S. Molecular classification of cancer: Class discovery and class prediction by gene expression monitoring. *Science* 286:531-537, 1999.

Goodman S. N., Zahurak M. L., and Piantadoosi S. Some practical improvements in the continual reassessment method for phase I studies. *Statisitics in Medicine* 14:1149–1161, 1995.

Gooley T., Martin P., Fisher L., and Pettinger M. Simulation as a design tool for Phase I/II clinical trials: An example from bone marrow transplantation. *Controlled Clinical Trials* 15:450–462, 1994.

Gooley T., Leissenring W., Crowley J., and Storer B. Estimation of failure probabilities in the presence of competing risks: New representations of old estimators. *Statistics in Medicine* 18:695-706, 1999.

Gordon R. *The Alarming History of Medicine*. New York: St. Martin's Press, 1993.

Gray R. J. A class of K-sample tests for comparing the cumulative incidence of a competing risk. *The Annals of Statistics* 16:1141–1154, 1988.

Green S. and Crowley J. Data monitoring committees for Southwest Oncology Group trials. *Statistics in Medicine* 12:451–455, 1993.

Green S. and Dahlberg S. Planned versus attained design in Phase II clinical trials. *Statistics in Medicine* 11:853–862, 1992.

Green S. J., Fleming T. R., and O'Fallon J. R. Policies for study monitoring and interim reporting of results. *Journal of Clinical Oncology* 5:1477–1484, 1987.

Green S. J., Fleming T. R., and Emerson S. Effects on overviews of early stopping rules for clinical trials. *Statistics in Medicine* 6:361–367, 1987.

Green S. Factorial designs with time to event endpoints. In *Handbook of Statistics in Clinical Oncology*, 2nd ed, J. Crowley and D. P. Ankerst (eds.). Boca Raton, FL: CRC Press, pp 181–190, 2006.

Green S. and Weiss G. Southwest Oncology Group standard response criteria, endpoint definitons and toxicity criteria. *Investigational New Drugs* 10:239–253, 1992.

Greipp P. R., San Miguel J., Durie B. G. M., Crowley J. J., Barlogie B., Blade J., Boccadoro M., et al. International staging system for multiple myeloma. *Journal of Clinical Oncology* 23:1–9, 2005.

Harrington D., Crowley J., George S., Pajak T., Redmond C., and Wieand S. The case against independent monitoring committees. *Statistics in Medicine* 13:1411–1414, 1994.

Harrington D., Fleming T., and Green S. Procedures for serial testing in censored survival data, in J. J. Crowley and R. A. Johnson (eds.) *Survival Analysis*. Hayward, CA: IMS Lecture Notes Monograph Series, 2:269–286, 1982.

Hawkins B. S. Data monitoring committees for multicenter clinical trials sponsored by the National Institutes of Health: Roles and membership of data monitoring committees for trials sponsored by the National Eye Institute. *Controlled Clinical Trials* 12:424–437, 1991.

Haybittle J. L. Repeated assessments of results in clinical trials of cancer treatment. *British Journal of Radiology* 44:793–797, 1971.

Heath E. I., LoRusso P. M., Ivy S. P., Rubinstein L., Christian M. C., and Heilbrun L. K. Theoretical and practical application of traditional and accelerated titration Phase I clinical trial designs: The Wayne State University experience. *Journal of Biopharmaceutical Statistics* 19:414–423, 2009.

Hellman S. and Hellman D. S. Of mice but not men: Problems of the randomized clinical trial. *New England Journal of Medicine* 324:1585–1589, 1991.

Henderson I. C., Hayes D., and Gelman R. Dose-response in the treatment of breast cancer: A critical review. *Journal of Clinical Oncology* 6:1501–1515, 1988.

Herbst R. S., Kelly K., Chansky K., Mack P. C., Franklin W. A., Hirsch F.R., Atkins J.N., et al. Phase II selection design of concurrent chemotherapy and cetuximab versus chemotherqapy followed by cetuximab in advanced-stage non-small-cell lung cancer: Southwest Oncology Study S0342. *Journal of Clinical Oncology* 28:4747–4754, 2010.

Hill A. B. Principles of Medical Statistics. London: *Lancet*, 1937.

Hill A. B. Memories of the British streptomycin trial in tuberculosis. *Controlled Clinical Trials* 11:77–79, 1990.

Hoering A., LeBlanc M., and Crowley J. Randomized phase III clinical trial designs for targeted agents. *Clinical Cancer Research* 14:4358–4367, 2008.

Hoering A., LeBlanc M., and Crowley J. Seamless phase I/II trial design for assessing toxicity and efficacy for targeted agents. *Clinical Cancer Research* 17:640–646, 2011.

Hogan J. W. and Laird N. M. Mixture models for the joint distribution of repeated measures and event times. *Statistics in Medicine* 16:239–257, 1997.

Horstmann E., McCabe M., Grochow L., Yamamoto S., Rubinstein L., Budd T., Shoemaker D., Emanuel E., and Grady C. Risks and benefits of Phase 1 oncology trials, 1991-2002. *New England Journal of Medicine* 352:895–904, 2005.

Hróbjartsson A., Forfang E., Haahr M., Als-Nielsen B., and Brorson S. Blinded trials taken to the test: An analysis of randomized clinical trials that report tests for the success of blinding. *International Journal of Epidemiology* 36:654–663, 2007.

Hryniuk W. and Levine M. N. Analysis of dose intensity for adjuvant chemotherapy trials in stage II breast cancer. *Journal of Clinical Oncology* 4:1162–1170, 1986.

Hsieh F.-Y., Crowley J., and Tormey D. C. Some test statistics for use in multistate survival analysis. *Biometrika* 70:111–119, 1983.

Huang B. and Chappell R. Three-dose-cohort designs in cancer phase I trials. *Statistics in Medicine* 27:2070–2093, 2008.

Huff D. *How to Lie with Statistics*. New York: Norton, 1954.

Hunsberger S., Rubinstein L. V., Dancey J., and Korn E. L. Dose escalation trial designs based on a molecularly targeted endpoint. *Statistics in Medicine* 24:2171–2181, 2005.

Hunsberger S., Zhao Y., and Simon R. A comparison of phase II study strategies. *Clinical Cancer Research* 15:5950–5955, 2009.

Inoue L. Y., Thall P. F., and Berry D. A. Seamlessly expanding a phase II trial to phase III. *Biometrics* 58:823–831, 2002.

ISIS-2 Collaborative Group. Randomized trial of intravenous streptokinase, oral aspirin, both, or neither among 17,187 cases of suspected acute myocardial infarction: ISIS-2. *Lancet* 332:349–60, 1988.

Ivanova A., Montazer-Haghighi A., Mohanty S. G., and Durham S. D. Improved up-and-down designs for phase I trials. *Statistics in Medicine* 22:69–82, 2003.

Jennison C. and Turnbull B. W. Confidence intervals for a binomial parameter following a multistage test with application to MIL-STD 105D and medical trials. *Technometrics* 25:49–58, 1983.

Jung S.-H. and Kim K. M. On the estimation of the binomial probability in multistage clinical trials. *Statistics in Medicine* 23:881–896, 2004.

Kalbfleisch J. D. and Prentice R. L. *The Statistical Analysis of Failure Time Data*. New York: Wiley, 1980.

Kaplan E. L. and Meier P. Nonparametric estimation from incomplete observations. *Journal of the American Statistical Association* 53:457–481, 1958.

Kassirer J. P. Clinical trials and meta-analysis: What they do for us. (editorial) *New England Journal of Medicine* 325:273–274, 1992.

Kelly K., Crowley J., Bunn P. A., Hazuka M., Beasley K., Upchurch C., Weiss G., et al. Role of recombinant interferon alfa-2a maintenance in patients with limited-stage small-cell lung cancer responding to concurrent chemoradiation: A Southwest Oncology Group study. *Journal of Clinical Oncology* 13:2924–2930, 1995.

Khan J., Wei J. S., Ringner M., Saal L. H., Ladanyi M., Westerman F., Berthold F., Schwab M., Antonescu C. R., Peterson C., and Meltzer P. S. Classification and diagnostic prediction of cancers using gene expression profiling and artificial neural networks. *Nature Medicine* 7:673–679, 2001.

Kies M. S., Mira J., Chen T., and Livingston R. B. Value of chest radiation therapy in limited small cell lung cancer after chemotherapy induced complete disease remission (for the Southwest Oncology Group). (abstract) *Proceedings of the American Society of Clinical Oncology* 1:141(C-546), 1982.

Kies M. S., Mira J., Crowley J., Chen T., Pazdur R., Grozea P., Rivkin S., Coltman C., Ward J. H., and Livingston R. B. Multimodal therapy for limited small cell lung cancer: A randomized study of induction combination chemotherapy with or without thoracic radiation in complete responders; and with wide field versus reduced-field radiation in partial responders: A Southwest Oncology Group study. *Journal of Clinical Oncology* 5:592–600, 1987.

Kieser M. and Friede T. Simple procedures for blinded sample size adjustment that do not affect the type I error rate. *Statistics in Medicine* 22:3571–3581, 2003.

Kim E. S., Herbst R. S., Wistuba I. I., Lee J. J., Blumenschein G. R. Jr., Tsao A., Stewart D. J., et al. The BATTLE trial: Personalizing therapy for lung cancer. *Cancer Discovery* 1:43–51, 2011.

Kindler H. L., Friberg G., Singh D. A., Locker G., Nattam S., Kozloff M., Taber D. A., et al. Phase II trial of bevacizumab plus gemcitabine in patients with advanced pancreatic cancer. *Journal of Clinical Oncology* 23:8033–8040, 2005.

Kindler H. L., Niedzwiecki D., Hollis D., Sutherland S., Schrag D., Hurwitz H., Innocenti F., et al. Gemcitabine plus bevacizumab compared with gemcitabine plus placebo in patients with advanced pancreatic cancer: Phase III trial of the Cancer and Leukemia Group B (CALGB 80303). *Journal of Clinical Oncology* 28:3617–3622, 2010.

Klimt C. R. Varied acceptance of clinical trial results. *Controlled Clinical Trials* 10 (Supplement):1355–1415, 1989.

Kopecky K. K. and Green S. Noninferiority trials. In *Handbook of Statistics in Clinical Oncology*, 2nd ed. J. Crowley and D. P. Ankerst (eds.). Boca Raton, FL: CRC Press, pp 191–206, 2006.

Korn E. L. and Friedlin B. Outcome-adpative randomization: Is it useful? *Joural of Clinical Oncology* 29:771–776, 2011.

Lamm D. L., Blumenstein B. A., Crawford E. D., Crissman J. D., Lowe B. A., Smith J. A., Sarosdy M. F., et al. Randomized intergroup comparison of bacillus Calmette-Guerin immunotherapy and mitomycin C chemotherapy prophylaxis in superficial transitional cell carcinoma of the bladder: A Southwest Oncology Group study. *Urologic Oncology* 1:119–126, 1995.

Lan K. and DeMets D. Changing frequency of interim analysis in sequential monitoring. *Biometrics* 45:1017–1020, 1989.

Lan K., Simon R., and Halperin, M. Stochastically curtailed test in long-term clinical trials. *Sequential Analysis* 1:207–219, 1982.

Lancaster H. O. *Quantitative Methods in Biological and Medical Sciences*. New York: Springer-Verlag, 1994.

Laurie J. A., Moertel C. G., Fleming T. R., Wieand H. S., Leigh J. E., Rubin J., McCormack G. W., et al. Surgical adjuvant therapy of large-bowel carcinoma: An evaluation of levamisole and the combination of levamisole and fluorouracil. *Journal of Clinical Oncology* 7:1447–1456, 1989.

LeBlanc M. and Crowley J. Relative risk trees for censored survival data. *Biometrics* 48:411–425, 1992.

LeBlanc M. and Crowley J. Survival trees by goodness of split. *Journal of the American Statistical Association* 88:457–467, 1993.

LeBlanc M., Jacobson J., and Crowley J. Partitioning and peeling for constructing prognostic groups. *Statistical Methods in Medical Research* 11:1–28, 2002.

LeBlanc M., Rankin C., and Crowley J. Multiple histology phase II trials. *Clinical Cancer Research* 15:4256–4262, 2009.

Lee J. and Tseng C. Uniform power method for sample size calculation in historical control studies with binary response. *Controlled Clinical Trials* 22:390–400, 2001.

Leichman C. G., Fleming T. R., Muggia F. M., Tangen C. M., Ardalan B., Doroshow J. H., Meyers F. J., et al. Phase II study of fluorouracil and its modulation in advanced colorectal cancer: A Southwest Oncology Group study. *Journal of Clinical Oncology* 13:1301–1311, 1995.

Lind J. *A Treatise of the Scurvy*. Edinburgh: Sands, Murray, and Cochran, 1753.

Lin X., Allred A., and Andrews G. A two-stage phase II trial design utilizing both primary and secondary endpoints. *Pharmaceutical Statistics* 7:88–92, 2008.

Liu P.-Y. and Dahlberg S. Design and analysis of multiarm clinical trials with survival endpoints. *Controlled Clinical Trials* 16:119–130, 1995.

Liu P.-Y., Dahlberg S., and Crowley J. Selection designs for pilot studies based on survival endpoints. *Biometrics* 49:391–398, 1993.

Liu P.-Y., Voelkel J., Crowley J., and Wolf M. Sufficient conditions for treatment responders to have longer survival than non-responders. *Statistics and Probability Letters* 18:205–208, 1993.

Liu P.-Y, Tsai W.-Y., and Wolf M. Design and analysis for survival data under order restrictions: A modified ordered logrank test. *Statistics in Medicine* 17:1469–79, 1998.

Liu P. Y., Moon J., and LeBlanc M. Phase II Selection designs. In *Handbook of Statistics in Clinical Oncology*, 2nd ed. J. Crowley and D. P. Ankerst (eds.) Boca Raton, FL: CRC Press, pp 155–166, 2006.

Liu Q. and Pledger G. Phase 2 and combination designs to accelerate drug development. *Journal of the American Statistical Association* 100:493–502, 2005.

Liver Infusion Meta-Analysis Group. Portal vein infusion of cytotoxic drugs after colorectal cancer surgery: A meta-analysis of 10 randomised studies involving 4000 patients. *Journal of the National Cancer Institute* 89:497–505, 1997.

London W. and Chang M. One- and two-stage designs for stratifed phase II clinical trials. *Statistics in Medicine* 24:2597–2611, 2005.

Louvet C., Lledo T. A., Hammel P., Bleiberg H., Bouleuc C., Gamelin E., Flesch M., Cvitkovic E., and de Gramont A. Gemcitabine combined with oxaliplatin in advanced pancreatic adenocarcinoma: Final results of a GERCOR multicenter phase II study. *Journal of Clinical Oncology* 20:1512–1518, 2002.

Louvet C., Labianca R., Hammel P., Lledo G., Zampino M. G., Andre A., Zaniboni A., et al. Gemcitabine in combination with oxaliplatin compared with gemcitabine alone in locally advanced or metastatic pancreatic cancer: Results of a GERCOR and GISCAD phase III trial. *Journal of Clinical Oncology* 23:3509–3516, 2005.

Macdonald J. S., Smalley, S. R., Benedetti J., Hundahl S. A., Estes N. C., Stemmerman G. N., Haller D. G., Ajani J. A., Gunderson L. L., Jessup J. M., and Martenson J. A. Chemoradiotherapy after surgery compared with surgery alone for adenocarcinoma of the stomach or gastroesophageal junction. *New England Journal of Medicine* 345:725–730, 2001.

Machtay M., Kaiser L. R., and Glatstein E. Is meta-analysis really meta-physics? *Chest* 116:539–544, 1999.

Mackillop W. J. and Johnston P. A. Ethical problems in clinical research: The need for empirical studies of the clinical trials process. *Journal of Chronic Diseases* 39:177–188, 1986.

Macklin R. The ethical problems with sham surgery in clinical research. *New England Journal of Medicine* 341:992–996, 1999.

Makuch R. and Simon R. Sample size consideration for non-randomized comparative studies. *Journal of Chronic Diseases* 33:175–181, 1980.

Mandrekar S. J. and Sargent D. J. Randomized phase II trials: Time for a new era in clinical trial design. *Journal of Thoracic Oncology* 5:932–934, 2010.

Mantel N. Evaluation of survival data and two new rank order statistics arising in its consideration. *Cancer Chemotherapy Reports* 50:163–170, 1966.

Margolin K. M., Green S., Osborne K., Doroshow J. H., Akman S. A., Leong L. A., Morgan R. J., et al. Phase II trial of 5-fluorouracil and high-dose folinic acid as first- or second-line therapy for advanced breast cancer. *American Journal of Clinical Oncology* 17:175–180, 1994.

Markman, Maurie. Letter to the editor. Serious ethical dilemma of single-agent pegylated liposomal doxorubicin employed as a control arm in ovarian cancer chemotherapy trials. *Journal of Clinical Oncology* 28:e319–e320, 2010.

Marubini E. and Valsecchi M. G. *Analysing Survival Data from Clinical Trials and Observational Studies*. New York: Wiley, 1995.

McCracken D., Janaki L. M., Crowley J., Taylor S. A., Giri P. G., Weiss G. B., Gordon J. W., Baker L. H., Mansouri A., and Kuebler J. P. Concurrent chemotherapy/radiotherapy for limited small-cell carcinoma: A Southwest Oncology Group study. *Journal of Clinical Oncology* 8:892–898, 1990.

McFadden E. T., LoPresti F., Bailey L. R., Clarke E., and Wilkins P. C. Approaches to data management. *Controlled Clinical Trials* 16:30S–65S, 1995.

Meier P. Statistics and medical experimentation. *Biometrics* 31:511–529, 1975.

Miller T. P., Crowley J., Mira J., Schwartz J. G., Hutchins L., Baker L., Natale R., Chase E. M., and Livingston R. A randomized trial of treatment of chemotherapy and radiotherapy for stage III non-small cell lung cancer. *Cancer Therapeutics* 1:229–236, 1998.

Mira J. G., Kies M. S., and Chen T. Influence of chest radiotherapy in response, remission duration, and survival in chemotherapy responders in localized small cell lung carcinoma: A Southwest Oncology Group Study. *Proceedings of the American Society of Clinical Oncology* 3:212 (C-827), 1984.

Moeller S. An extension of the continual reassessment methods using a preliminary up-and-down design in a dose finding study in cancer patients, in order to investigate a greater range of doses. *Statistics in Medicine* 14:911–922, 1995.

Moertel C. G., Fleming T. R., MacDonald J. S., Haller D. G., Laurie J. A., Goodman P. J., Ungerleider J. S., et al. Levamisole and fluorouracil for adjuvant therapy of resected colon carcinoma. *New England Journal of Medicine* 322:352–358, 1990.

Moher D., Hopewell S., Schulz K. F., Montori V., Gøtzsche P. C., Devereaux P. J., Elbourne D., Egger M., and Altman D. G. for the CONSORT Group. CONSORT 2010 Explanation and elaboration: Updated guidelines for reporting parallel group randomised trial. *British Medical Journal* 340:c869, 2010.

Moinpour C., Feigl P., Metch B., Hayden K., Meyskens F., and Crowley J. Quality of life end points in cancer clinical trials: Review and recommendations. *Journal of the National Cancer Institute* 81:485–496, 1989.

Moinpour C. M. Costs of quality of life research in Southwest Oncology Group trials. *Monographs of the Journal of the National Cancer Institute* 20:11–16, 1996.

Moinpour C., Triplett J., McKnight B., Lovato l., Upchurch C., Leichman C., Muggia F., et al. Challenges posed by non-random missing quality of life data in an advanced stage colorectal cancer clinical trial. *Psycho-Oncology* 9:340–354, 2000.

Monro A. Collections of blood in cancerous breasts. In Monro A. *The Works of Alexander Monro*. Edinburgh: Ch Elliot, 1781.

Norfolk D., Child J. A., Cooper E. H., Kerrulsh S., and Milford-Ward A. Serum β_2 microglobulin in myelomatosis: Potential value in stratification and monitoring. *British Journal of Cancer* 42:510–515, 1980.

O'Brien P. Procedures for comparing samples with multiple endpoints. *Biometrics* 40:1079–1087, 1984.

Olanow C. W., Goetz C., Kordower J., Stoessl A. J., Sossi V, Brin M., Shannon K., et al. A double-blind controlled trial of bilateral fetal nigral transplantation in Parkinson's disease. *Annals of Neurology* 54:403–414, 2003.

O'Malley J., Normand S.-L., and Kuntz R. Sample size calculation for a historically controlled clinical trial with adjustment for covariates. *Journal of Biopharmaceutical Statistics* 12:227–247, 2002.

O'Quigley J., Pepe M., and Fisher L. Continual reassessment method: A practical design for Phase I clinical trials. *Biometrics* 46:33–48, 1990.

O'Quigley J., Hughes M., and Fenton T. Dose-finding for HIV studies. *Biometrics* 57:1018–1029, 2001.

O'Quigley J. Dose finding designs using continual reassessment methods. In *Handbook of Statistics in Clinical Oncology*, 3rd ed., Crowley J. and Hoering A. (eds.) New York: Marcel Dekker, 2011.

Panageas K., Smith A., Gönen M., and Chapman P. An optimal two-stage phase II design utilizing complete and partial response information separately. *Controlled Clinical Trials* 23:367–379, 2002.

Passamani E. Clinical trials—are they ethical? *New England Journal of Medicine* 324:1589–1592, 1991.

Pater J. and Crowley J. Sequential randomization. In *Handbook of Statistics in Clinical Oncology*, 2nd ed. J. Crowley and D. P. Ankerst, (eds.). Boca Raton, FL: CRC Press, pp 589–596, 2006.

Penel N., Isambert N., Leblond P., Ferte C., Duhamel A., and Bonneterre J. "Classical 3 + 3 design" versus "accelerated titration designs": Analysis of 270 phase 1 trials investigating anti-cancer agents. *Investigational New Drugs* 27:552–556, 2009.

Permutt T. Testing for imbalance of covariates in controlled experiments. *Statistics in Medicine* 9:1455–1462, 1990.

Pérol M., Léna H., Thomas P., Robinet G., Fournel P., Coste E., Belleguic C., et al. Phase II randomized multicenter study evaluating a treatment regimen alternating docetaxel and cisplatin–vinorelbine with a cisplatin–vinorelbine control group in patients with stage IV non-small-cell lung cancer: GFPC 97.01 study. *Annals of Oncology* 13:742–747, 2002.

Peterson B. and George S. L. Sample size requirements and length of study for testing interaction in a $2 \times k$ factorial design when time to failure is the outcome. *Controlled Clinical Trials* 14:511–522, 1993.

Peto R. and Peto J. Asymptotically efficient rank invariant test procedures. *Journal of the Royal Statistical Society, Series A* 135:185–198, 1972.

Peto R., Pike M. C., Armitage P., Breslow N. E., Cox D. R., Howard S. V., Mantel N., McPherson K., Peto J., and Smith P. G. Design and analysis of randomized clinical trials requiring prolonged observation of each patient. I. Introduction and design. *British Journal of Cancer* 34:585–612, 1976.

Philip P. A., Benedetti J., Corless C. L., Wong R., O'Reilly E. M., Flynn P. J., Rowland K. M., et al. Phase III study comparing gemcitabine plus cetuximab versus gemcitabine in patients with advanced pancreatic adenocarcinoma: Southwest Oncology Group–Directed intergroup trial S0205. *Journal of Clinical Oncology* 28:3605–3610, 2010.

Piantadosi S. *Clinical Trials: A Methodological Perspective.* Hoboken, NJ: Wiley, 2005.

Pocock S. J. and Simon R. Sequential treatment assignment with balancing for prognostic factors in the controlled clinical trial. *Biometrics* 31:348–361, 1975.

Poplin E., Feng Y., Berlin J., Rothenberg M. L., Hochster H., Mitchell E., Alberts S., et al. Phase III, randomized study of gemcitabine and oxaliplatin versus gemcitabine (fixed-dose rate infusion) compared with gemcitabine (30-minute infustion) in patients with pancreatic carcinoma E6201: A trial of the Eastern Cooperative Oncology Group. *Journal of Clinical Oncology* 27:3778–3785, 2009.

Prentice R. L. Linear rank tests with right censored data. *Biometrika* 65:167–179, 1978.

Prentice R. L., Kalbfleisch J. D., Peterson A. V. Jr., Flournoy N., Farewell V. T., and Breslow N. E. The analysis of failure times in the presence of competing risks. *Biometrics* 34:541–554, 1978.

Prentice R. L. Surrogate endpoints in clinical trials: Discussion, definition and operational criteria. *Statistics in Medicine* 8:431–440, 1989.

Pritza D. R., Bierman M. H., and Hammeke M. D. Acute toxic effects of sustained-release verapamil in chronic renal failure. *Archives of Internal Medicine* 151:2081–2084, 1991.

Quackenbush J. Computational analysis of microarray data. *Nature Reviews* 2:418–427, 2001.

Redman M. and Crowley J. Small randomized trials. *Journal of Thoracic Oncology* 2:1–2, 2007.

Redman M. Early stopping of clinical trials. In *Handbook of Statistics in Clinical Oncology*. J. Crowley and A. Hoering (eds.). Boca Raton, FL: Chapman and Hall/CRC Press, 2012.

Redmond C., Fisher B., and Wieand H. S. The methodologic dilemma in retrospectively correlating the amount of chemotherapy received in adjuvant therapy protocols with disease-free survival. *Cancer Treatment Reports* 67:519–526, 1983.

Rivkin S. E., Green S., Metch B., Glucksberg H., Gad-el-Mawla N., Constanzi J. J., Hoogstraten B., et al. Adjuvant CMFVP versus melphalan for operable breast cancer with positive axillary nodes: 10-year results of a Southwest Oncology Group study. *Journal of Clinical Oncology* 7:1229–1238, 1989.

Rivkin S. E., Green S., Metch B., Jewell W., Costanzi J., Altman S., Minton J., O'Bryan R., and Osborne C. K. One versus 2 years of CMFVP adjuvant chemotherapy in axillary node-positive and estrogen receptor negative patients: A Southwest Oncology Group study. *Journal of Cinical Oncology* 11:1710–1716, 1993.

Rivkin S. E., Green S., Metch B., Cruz A. B., Abeloff A. M., Jewell W. R., Costanzi J. J., Farrar W. B., Minton J. P., and Osborne C. K. Adjuvant CMFVP versus tamoxifen versus concurrent CMFVP and tamoxifen for postmenopausal, node-positive and estrogen-receptor positive breast cancer patients: A Southwest Oncology Group study. *Journal of Clinical Oncology* 12:2078–2085, 1994.

Rivkin S. E., Green S., O'Sullivan J., Cruz A., Abeloff M. D., Jewell W. R., Costanzi J. J., Farra W. B., and Osborne C. K. Adjuvant CMFVP plus ovariechtomy for premenopausal, node-positive and estrogen receptor-positive breast cancer patients: A Southwest Oncology Group study. *Journal of Clinical Oncology* 14:46–51, 1996.

Rockhold F. W. and Enas G. G. Data monitoring and interim analysis in the pharmaceutical industry: Ethical and logistical considerations. *Statistics in Medicine* 12:471–479, 1993.

Rosner B. *Fundamentals of Biostatistics*, 2nd ed. Boston: Duxbury, 1986.

Rothwell P. Subgroup analysis in randomized controlled trials: Importance, indications and interpretation. *Lancet* 365:176–186, 2005.

Royall R. Ethics and statistics in randomized clinical trials. *Statistical Science* 6:52–88, 1991.

Royston P., Parmar M. K. B., and Qian W. Novel designs for multi-arm clinical trials with survival outcomes with an application in ovarian cancer. *Statististics in Medicine* 22:2239–2256, 2003.

Rubinstein L. V., Korn E. L., Friedlin B., Hunsberger S., Ivy S. P., and Smith M. A. Design issues of randomized phase II trials and a proposal for phase II screening trials. *Journal of Clinical Oncology* 23:7199–7206, 2005.

Rubinstein L. V., Crowley J., Ivy P., LeBlanc M., and Sargent D. J. Randomized phase II designs. *Clinical Cancer Research* 15:1883–1890, 2009.

Salmon S. E., Haut A., Bonnet J. D., Amare M., Weick J. K., Durie B. G. M., and Dixon D. O. Alternating combination chemotherapy and levamisole improves survival in multiple myeloma: A Southwest Oncology Group study. *Journal of Clinical Oncology* 1:453–461, 1983.

Salmon S. E., Tesh D., Crowley J., Saeed S., Finley P., Milder M. S., Hutchins L. F., et al. Chemotherapy is superior to sequential hemibody irradiation for remission consolidation in multiple myeloma: A Southwest Oncology Group study. *Journal of Clinical Oncology* 8:1575–1584, 1990.

Salmon S. E., Crowley J., Grogan T. M., Finley P., Pugh R. P., and Barlogie B. Combination chemotherapy, glucocorticoids, and interferon alpha in the treatment of multiple myeloma: A Southwest Oncology Group study. *Journal of Clinical Oncology* 12:2405–2414, 1994.

Salmon S. E., Crowley J. J., Balcerzak S. P., Roach P. W., Taylor S. A., Rivkin S. E., and Samlowski W. Interferon versus interferon plus prednisone remission maintenance therapy for multiple myeloma: A Southwest Oncology Group study. *Journal of Clinical Oncology* 16:890–896, 1998.

Sargent D. F., Wieand S., Haller D. G., Gray R., Benedetti J., Buyse M., Labianca R., et al. Disease-free survival versus overall survival as a primary end point for adjuvant colon cancer studies: Individual patient data from 20,898 patients on 18 randomized trials. *Journal of Clinical Oncology* 23:8664–8670, 2005.

Sargent D. J., Conley B. A., Allegra C., and Collette L. Clinical trial designs for predictive marker validation in cancer treatment trials. *Journal of Clinical Oncology* 9:2020–2027, 2005.

Sasieni P. D. and Winnett A. Graphical approaches to exploring the effects of prognostic factors on survival. In *Handbook of Statistics in Clinical Oncology*, 1st edition. J. Crowley (ed.). Boca Raton, FL: Chapman and Hall/CRC Press, pp 433–456, 2001.

Schaid D., Wieand S., and Therneau T. Optimal two-stage screening designs for survival comparisons. *Biometrika* 77:507–513, 1990.

Schemper M. and Smith T. L. A note on quantifying follow-up in studies of failure time. *Controlled Clinical Trials* 17:343–346, 1996.

Schoenfeld D. Sample-size formula for the proportional-hazards regression model. *Biometrics* 39:499–503, 1983.

Schulz K. F., Altman D. G., and Moher D. for the CONSORT Group. CONSORT 2010 Statement: Updated guidelines for reporting parallel group randomised trials. *British Medical Journal* 340:c332, 2010.

Schumacher M., Holländer N., Schwarzer G., and Sauerbrei W. Prognostic factor studies. In *Handbook of Statistics in Clinical Oncology*, 2nd edition. J. Crowley and D. P. Ankerst, (eds.). Boca Raton, FL: Chapman and Hall/CRC Press, pp 289–334, 2006.

Segal M. R. Regression trees for censored data. *Biometrics* 44:35–48, 1988.

Sessa C., Capri G., Gianni L., Peccatori F., Grasselli G., Bauer J., Zucchetti M., et al. Clinical and pharmacological phase I study with accelerated titration design of a daily times five schedule of BBR3436, a novel cationic triplatinum complex. *Annals of Oncology* 11:977–983, 2000.

Shapiro A. and Shapiro K. *The Powerful Placebo: From Ancient Priest to Modern Physician*. Baltimore, MD: Johns Hopkins University Press, 1997.

Shepherd F. A., Pereira J., Ciuleanu T. E., Tan E. H., Hirsh V., Thongprasert S., Campos D., et al. for the National Cancer Institute of Canada Clinical Trials Group. Erlotinib in previously treated non-small-cell lung cancer. *New England Journal of Medicine* 353:123–132, 2005.

Silverman W. A. and Chalmers I. Sir Austin Bradford Hill: An appreciation. *Controlled Clinical Trials* 13:100–105, 1991.

Silverman W. A. Doctoring: From art to engineering. *Controlled Clinical Trials* 13:97–99, 1992.

Simon R. and Wittes R. E. Methodologic guidelines for reports of clinical trials. (editorial) *Cancer Treatment Reports* 69:1–3, 1985.

Simon R. How large should a Phase II trial of a new drug be? *Cancer Treatment Reports* 71:1079–1085, 1987.

Simon R. Optimal two-stage designs for Phase II clinical trials. *Controlled Clinical Trials* 10:1–10, 1989.

Simon R. Practical aspects of interim monitoring of clinical trials. *Statistics in Medicine* 13:1401–1409, 1994.

Simon R. and Ungerleider R. Memorandum to Cooperative Group Chairs, 1992.

Simon R., Wittes R., and Ellenberg S. Randomized Phase II clinical trials. *Cancer Treatment Reports* 69:1375–1381, 1985.

Simon R., Friedlin B., Rubenstein L., Arbuck S., Collins J., and Christian M. Accelerated titration designs for phase I clinical trials in oncology. *Journal of the National Cancer Institute* 89:1138–1147, 1997.

Simon R. and Maitournam A. Evaluating the efficiency of targeted designs for randomized clinical trials. *Clinical Cancer Research* 10:6759–6763, 2004.

Slamon D. J., Leyland-Jones B., Shak S., Fuchs H., Paton V., Bajamonde A., Fleming T., et al. Use of chemotherapy plus a monoclonal antibody against HER2 for metastatic breast cancer that overexpresses HER2. *New England Journal of Medicine* 344:783–792, 2001.

Slud E. Analysis of factorial survival experiments. *Biometrics* 50:25–38, 1994.

Smith J. *Patenting the Sun: Polio and the Salk Vaccine*. New York: William Morrow, 1990.

Smith J. S. Remembering the role of Thomas Francis, Jr. in the design of the 1954 Salk vaccine trial. *Controlled Clinical Trials* 13:181–184, 1992.

Spiegelhalter D. J., Freedman L. S., and Blackburn P. R. Monitoring clinical trials: Conditional or predictive power? *Controlled Clinical Trials* 7:8–17, 1986.

Sposto R. and Gaynon P. An adjustment for patient heterogeneity in the design of two-stage phase II trials. *Statistics in Medicine* 28:2566–2579, 2009.

Stallard N. and Todd S. Sequential designs for phase III clinical trials incorporating treatment selection. *Statistics in Medicine* 22:689–703, 2003.

Stewart David J., Whitney Simon N., and Kurzrock Razelle. Equipoise lost: Ethics, costs, and the regulation of cancer clinical research. *Journal of Clinical Oncology* 28:2925–2935, 2010.

Storer B. Design and analysis of Phase I clinical trials. *Biometrics* 45:925–938, 1989.

Storer B. Choosing a Phase I design. In *Handbook of Statistics in Clinical Oncology*, 3rd ed. J. Crowley and A. Hoering (eds.). New York: Marcel Dekker, 2011.

Stuart C. P. and Guthrie D. (eds.). *Lind's Treatise on Scurvy*. Edinburgh: University Press, 1953.

Stuart K. E., Hajdenberg A., Cohn A., Loh K. K., Miller W., White C., and Clendinnin N. J. A phase II trial of Thymitaq^{TM} (AG337) in patients with hepatocellular carcinoma (HCC). *Proceedings of the American Society of Clinical Oncology* 15:202 (#449), 1996.

Tang D.-I., Gnecco C., and Geller N. Design of group sequential clinical trials with multiple endpoints. *Journal of the American Statistical Association* 84:776–779, 1989.

Tang H., Foster N. R., Grothey A., Ansell S. M., Goldberg R. M., and Sargent D. J. Comparison of error rates in single-arm versus randomized phase II cancer clinical trials. *Journal of Clinical Oncology* 28:1936–1941, 2009.

Tangen C. M. and Crowley J. Phase II trials using time-to-event endpoints. In *Handbook of Statistics in Clinical Oncology*, 2nd ed. J. Crowley and D. P. Ankerst (eds.). Boca Raton, FL: CRC Press, pp 143–154, 2006.

Taube S. E., Jacobson J. W., and Lively T. G. Cancer diagnostics: Decision criteria for marker utilization in the clinic. *American Journal of Pharmacogenomics* 5:357–364, 2005.

Taylor I., Rowling J., and West C. Adjuvant cytotoxic liver perfusion for colorectal cancer. *British Journal of Surgery* 66:833–837, 1979.

Taylor I., Machin D., and Mullee M. A randomized controlled trial of adjuvant portal vein cytotoxic perfusion in colorectal cancer. *British Journal of Surgery* 72:359–363, 1985.

Taylor J. M., Braun T. M., and Li Z. Comparing an experimental agent to a standard agent: Relative merits of a one-arm or randomized two-arm Phase II design. *Clinical Trials* 3:335–348, 2006.

Thall P., Simon R., and Ellenberg S. Two-stage selection and testing designs for comparative clinical trials. *Biometrika* 75:303–310, 1988.

Thall P. F. and Estey E. H. Graphical methods for evaluating covariate effects in the Cox model. In *Handbook of Statistics in Clinical Oncology*, 1st edition. J. Crowley (ed.). Boca Raton, FL: Chapman and Hall/CRC Press, pp 411–432, 2001.

Thall P. F. and Russell K. E. A strategy for dose-finding and safety monitoring based on efficacy and adverse outcomes in phase I/II clinical trials. *Biometrics* 54:251–264, 1998.

Thall P. and Cook J. Dose-finding based on efficacy-toxicity trade-offs. *Biometrics* 60:684–693, 2004.

Thall P., Cook J., and Estey E. Adaptive dose selection using efficacy-toxicity trade-offs: Illustrations and practical considerations. *Journal of Biopharmaceutical Statistics* 16:623–638, 2006.

Thall P. F., Wathen K. J., Bekele B. N., Champlin R. E., Baker L. O., and Benjamin R. S. Hierarchical Bayesian approaches to phase II trials in diseases with multiple subtypes. *Statistics in Medicine* 22:763–780, 2003.

Therasse P., Arbuck S., Eisenhauer E., Wanders J., Kaplan R., Rubenstein L., Verweij J., et al. New guidelines to evaluate the response to treatment in solid tumors. *Journal of the National Cancer Institute* 92:205–216, 2000.

Therneau T. M. How many stratification factors are "too many" to use in a randomization plan? *Controlled Clinical Trials* 14:98–108, 1993.

Thomas L. *The Youngest Science*. New York: Viking Press, 1983.

Tibshirani R. J. and Hastie T. Local likelihood estimation. *Journal of the American Statistical Association* 82:559–567, 1987.

Tighiouart M., Rogatko A., and Babb J. S. Flexible Bayesian methods for cancer phase I clinical trials. Dose escalation with overdose control. *Statistics in Medicine* 24:2183–2196, 2005.

Troxel A. B., Harrington D. P., and Lipsitz S. R. Analysis of longitudinal data with non-ignorable non-monotone missing values. *Applied Statistics* 47:425–438, 1998.

Tsiatis A. and Mehta C. On the inefficiency of the adaptive design for monitoring clinical trials. *Biometrika* 90:367–378, 2003.

Ulm K., Seebauer M., Eberle S., Reck M., and Hessler S. Statistical methods to identify predictive factors. In *Handbook of Statistics in Clinical Oncology*, 2nd edition. J. Crowley and D. P. Ankerst, (eds.). Boca Raton, FL: Chapman and Hall/CRC Press, pp 335–346, 2006.

Vermorken J., Trigo R., Koralweski P., Diaz-Rubio E., Rolland F., Knecht R., Amellal N., Schueler A., and Baselga J. Open-label, uncontrolled, multicenter Phase II study to evaluate the efficacy and toxicity of cetuximab as a single agent in patients with recurrent and/or metastatic squamous cell carcinoma of the head and neck who failed to respond to platinum-based therapy. *Journal of Clinical Oncology* 25:2171–2177, 2007.

Volberding P. A., Lagakos S. W., Koch M. A., and the AIDS Clinical Trials Group of the National Institute of Allergy and Infectious Disease. Zidovudine in asymptomatic human immunodeficiency virus infection. *New England Journal of Medicine* 322:941–949, 1990.

Walters L. Data monitoring committees: The moral case for maximum feasible independence. *Statistics in Medicine* 12:575–580, 1993.

Wang R., Lagakos S., and Ware J. Statistics in medicine—reporting of subgroup analyses in clinical trials. *New England Journal of Medicine* 357:2189–2194, 2007.

Weick J. K., Kopecky K. J., Appelbaum F. R., Head D. R., Kingsbury L. L., Balcerzak S. P., Mills G. M., et al. A randomized investigation of high-dose versus standard dose cytosine arabinoside with daunorubicin in patients with previously untreated acute myeloid leukemia: A Southwest Oncology Group study. *Blood* 88:2841–2851, 1996.

Wei L. J. and Durham S. The randomized play-the-winner rule in medical trials. *Journal of the American Statistical Association* 73:830–843, 1978.

Weir C. J. and Lees K. R. Comparison of stratification and adaptive methods for treatment allocation in an acute stroke clinical trial. *Statistics in Medicine* 22:705–726, 2003.

Wolff J. *Lehre von den Krebskrankheiten von den ältesten Zeiten bis zur Gegenwart.* 4 Teile in 5Bde.Jena: G Fischer, 1907–1928.

Wolmark N., Rockette H., and Wickerham D. L. Adjuvant therapy of Dukes' A, B and C adenocarcinoma of the colon with portal-vein fluorouracil hepatic infusion: Preliminary results of National Surgical Adjuvant Breast and Bowel Project C-02. *Journal of Clinical Oncology* 8:1466–1475, 1990.

Wolmark N., Rockette H., and Fisher B. Adjuvant therapy for carcinoma of the colon: A review of NSABP clinical trial. In Salmon S. (ed). *Adjuvant Therapy of Cancer.* vol 7. Lippincott, pp 300–307, 1993.

World Medical Association General Assembly. World Medical Association Declaration of Helsinki: Ethical principles for medical research involving human subjects. *Journal of Internationale Bioethique* 15:124–129, 2004.

Xiong H. Q., Rosenberg A., LoBuglio A., Schmidt W., Wolff W. S., Deutsch J., Needle M., and Abbruzzese J. L. Cetuximab, a monoclonal antibody targeting the epidermal growth factor receptor, in combination with gemcitabine for advanced pancreatic cancer: A multicenter Phase II trial. *Journal of Clinical Oncology* 22:2610–2616, 2004.

Zee B., Melnychuck D., Dancey J., and Eisenhauer E. Multinomial Phase II cancer trials incorporating response and early progression. *Journal of Biopharmaceutical Statistics* 9:351–363, 1999.

Zelen M. A new design for randomized clinical trials. *New England Journal of Medicine* 300:1242–1246, 1979.

Zhan F., Hardin J., Bumm K., Zheng M., Tiand E., Wilson E., Crowley J., Barlogie B., and Shaughnessy J. Molecular profiling of multiple myeloma. *Blood* 99:1745–1757, 2002.

Zhang W., Sargent D., and Mandrekar S. An adaptive dose-finding design incorporating both toxicity and efficacy. *Statistics in Medicine* 25:2365–2383, 2006.

Zia M., Siu L., Pond G., and Chen E. Comparison of outcomes of Phase II studies and subsequent randomized control studies using identical chemotherapy regimens. *Journal of Clinical Oncology* 23:6982–6991, 2005.

Zubrod C. G., Schneiderman M., Frei M. III, Brindley C., Gold L., Shnider B., Oviedo R., Gorman J., Jones R. Jr., Jonsson U., Colsky J., Chalmers T., Ferguson B., Dederick M., Holland J., Selawry O., Regelson W., Lasagna L., and Owens A. H. Jr. Appraisal of methods for the study of chemotherapy of cancer in man: Comparative therapeutic trial of nitrogen mustard and thiophosphoramide. *Journal of Chronic Diseases* 11:7–33, 1960.

Zubrod C. G. Clinical trials in cancer patients: An introduction. *Controlled Clinical Trials* 3:185–187, 1982.

Index

Printed in the United States
by Baker & Taylor Publisher Services